T0212118

Lecture Notes in Computer Science　11840

More information about this series at http://www.springer.com/series/7412

Hayit Greenspan · Ryutaro Tanno ·
Marius Erdt et al. (Eds.)

Uncertainty for Safe Utilization of Machine Learning in Medical Imaging and Clinical Image-Based Procedures

First International Workshop, UNSURE 2019
and 8th International Workshop, CLIP 2019
Held in Conjunction with MICCAI 2019
Shenzhen, China, October 17, 2019
Proceedings

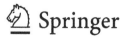 Springer

Editors
Hayit Greenspan
Tel Aviv University
Tel Aviv, Israel

Ryutaro Tanno
University College London
London, UK

Marius Erdt ⓘ
Fraunhofer Singapore
Nanyang Technological University
Singapore, Singapore

Additional Workshop Editors *see next page*

ISSN 0302-9743   ISSN 1611-3349   (electronic)
Lecture Notes in Computer Science
ISBN 978-3-030-32688-3   ISBN 978-3-030-32689-0   (eBook)
https://doi.org/10.1007/978-3-030-32689-0

LNCS Sublibrary: SL6 – Image Processing, Computer Vision, Pattern Recognition, and Graphics

This Springer imprint is published by the registered company Springer Nature Switzerland AG
The registered company address is: Gewerbestrasse 11, 6330 Cham, Switzerland

Additional Workshop Editors

Satellite Events Chair

Kenji Suzuki
Tokyo Institute of Technology
Yokohama, Japan

Workshop Chairs

Hongen Liao
Tsinghua University
Beijing, China

Hayit Greenspan
Tel Aviv University
Tel Aviv, Israel

Challenge Chairs

Qian Wang
Shanghai Jiaotong University
Shanghai, China

Bram van Ginneken
Radboud University
Nijmegen, The Netherlands

Tutorial Chair

Luping Zhou
University of Sydney
Sydney, Australia

International Workshop on Uncertainty for Safe Utilization of Machine Learning in Medical Imaging, UNSURE 2019

Tal Arbel
McGill University
Montreal, QC, Canada

Christian Baumgartner
ETH Zürich
Zürich, Switzerland

Adrian Dalca (iD)
Massachusetts Institute of Technology
Harvard Medical School
Cambridge, MA, USA

Carole H. Sudre
King's College London
University College London
London, UK

Ryutaro Tanno
University College London
London, UK

William M. Wells
Harvard Medical School
Boston, MA, USA

International Workshop on Clinical Image-Based Procedures, CLIP 2019

Klaus Drechsler
Aachen University of Applied Sciences
Aachen, Germany

Marius George Linguraru ⓘ
Children's National Healthcare System
Washington, D.C., USA

Raj Shekhar
Children's National Healthcare System
Washington, D.C., USA

Miguel Ángel González Ballester
ICREA - Universitat Pompeu Fabra
Barcelona, Spain

Marius Erdt
Fraunhofer Singapore, Singapore

Cristina Oyarzun Laura
Fraunhofer IGD
Darmstadt, Germany

Stefan Wesarg
Fraunhofer IGD
Darmstadt, Germany

Preface

UNSURE 2019 is the first workshop on Uncertainty for Safe Utilization of machine Learning in Medical imaging organized as a satellite event of the 22nd International Conference on Medical Image Computing and Computer Assisted Intervention (MICCAI 2019) in Shenzhen, China.

With the rise of machine learning techniques in medical imaging applications, the need to understand and acknowledge the limitations of a given technique has recently attracted the attention of the MICCAI community. The workshop aims to develop awareness and encourage research in the field of uncertainty modeling to enable safe implementation of machine learning tools in the clinical world.

The proceedings of UNSURE 2019 contain 8 high-quality papers of 8 to 10 pages selected among a pool of 15 submissions following a double-blind review process. Each submission was reviewed by 3 members of the Program Committee that gathered 21 experts in the applications of deep learning and Bayesian modeling to medical imaging.

The accepted papers cover the fields of uncertainty quantification and modeling as well as robustness to domain shift in deep learning settings with applications ranging from lesion detection and classification to registration, including intra-operative multispectral imaging.

In addition to the papers presented in the proceedings, the workshop welcomed two keynote presentations, from experts Dr. Koen Van Leemput (Harvard Medical School, USA) and Dr. Yinzheng Li (Microsoft Research Cambridge, UK).

We hope this workshop has highlighted both theoretical and practical challenges in communicating uncertainties and further encourages research to (a) improve safety in the application of machine learning tools and (b) assist in the translation of such tools to clinical practice.

We would like to thank all the authors for submitting their manuscripts to UNSURE, as well as the Program Committee members for the quality of their feedback and dedication to the review process.

August 2019

Tal Arbel
Christian Baumgartner
Adrian Dalca
Carole H. Sudre
Ryutaro Tanno
William M. Wells

Organization

Program Committee Chairs

Tal Arbel   McGill University, Canada
Christian Baumgartner   ETH Zürich, Switzerland
Adrian Dalca   Harvard Medical School and Massachusetts Institute of Technology, USA
Carole H. Sudre   King's College London, UK
Ryutaro Tanno   University College London, UK
William M. Wells   Harvard Medical School, USA

Program Committee

Felix Bragman   King's College London, UK
Liane Canas   King's College London, UK
M. Jorge Cardoso   King's College London, UK
Juan Cerrolaza   Accenture, UK
Daniel Coelho de Castro   Imperial College London, UK
Reuben Dorent   King's College London, UK
Zach Eaton-Rosen   King's College London, UK
Lucas Fidon   King's College London, UK
Angelos Filos   Oxford University, UK
Alejandro Granados   King's College London, UK
Juan Eugenio Iglesias   Harvard Medical School, USA
Leo Joskowicz   Hebrew University of Jerusalem, Israel
Simon Kohl   Karlsruhe Institute of Technology, Germany
Hongxiang Lin   University College London, UK
Raghav Mehta   McGill University, Canada
Tanya Nair   McGill University, Canada
Kerem Can Tezcan   ETH Zürich, Switzerland
Koen Van Leemput   Harvard Medical School, USA
Thomas Varsavsky   King's College London, UK
Christian Wachinger   Ludwig Maximilian University Munich, Germany
Daniel Worrall   University of Amsterdam, The Netherlands

Preface

On October 17, 2019, the 8th International Workshop on Clinical Image-based Procedures: From Planning to Intervention (CLIP 2019) was held in Shenzhen, China in conjunction with the 22nd International Conference on Medical Image Computing and Computer Assisted Intervention (MICCAI 2019). Following the tradition set in the last seven years, this year's edition of the workshop was an exciting forum for the discussion and dissemination of clinically tested, state-of-the-art methods for image-based planning, monitoring, and evaluation of medical procedures.

Nowadays, it has become more and more important for many clinical applications to base decisions not only on image data alone, thus a focus of CLIP 2019 was the creation of holistic patient models. Here, image data such as radiologic images, microscopy images, and photographs are combined with non-image information such as 'omics' data (e.g. genomics, proteomics), lifestyle data, demographics, EEG, and others to build a more complete picture of the individual patient and to subsequently provide better diagnosis and therapies.

CLIP 2019 provided a forum for work centered on specific clinical applications, including techniques and procedures based on comprehensive clinical image and other data. Submissions related to applications already in use and evaluated by clinical users were particularly encouraged. Furthermore, novel techniques and applications that are looking at combining image analysis with clinical data mining and analytics, user studies, and other heterogeneous data were a focus as well.

In CLIP's 8th edition, world-class researchers and clinicians came together to present ways to strengthen links between computer scientists and engineers, and surgeons, interventional radiologists, and radiation oncologists.

In 2019, CLIP received 15 original manuscripts from all over the world. Each of the manuscripts underwent a meticulous double-blind peer-review by at least three members of the Program Committee, all of them prestigious experts in the field of medical image analysis and clinical translations of technology. 11 manuscripts were accepted for oral presentation at the workshop.

In addition to the presentation of high-quality papers, a highlight of CLIP has always been the keynotes featuring prominent experts in the field. This year, Dr. Chen Hao, founder and CEO of Imsight Medical Technology shared his experience in founding a company in the medical image analysis domain and translating latest research to the market.

We would like to thank our Program Committee for its invaluable contributions and continuous support of CLIP over the years. Finding spare time in busy schedules and during holiday season is not an easy task and we are very grateful to all our members as CLIP 2019 would not have been possible without them. We would also like to thank all authors for their high-quality contributions this year as well as their efforts to make CLIP 2019 a success. Finally, we would like to thank all MICCAI 2019 organizers and team for supporting the organization of CLIP 2019.

October 2019

Marius Erdt
Klaus Drechsler
Marius George Linguraru
Cristina Oyarzun Laura
Raj Shekhar
Stefan Wesarg
Miguel Ángel González Ballester

Organization

Organizing Committee

Klaus Drechsler — Aachen University of Applied Sciences, Germany
Marius Erdt — Fraunhofer Singapore, Singapore
Miguel González Ballester — ICREA – Universitat Pompeu Fabra, Spain
Marius George Linguraru — Children's National Healthcare System, USA
Cristina Oyarzun Laura — Fraunhofer IGD, Germany
Raj Shekhar — Children's National Healthcare System, USA
Stefan Wesarg — Fraunhofer IGD, Germany

Program Committee

Mario Ceresa
Juan Cerrolaza
Yufei Chen
Chaoqun Dong
Alexander Distergoft
Camila Gonzalez
Jan Egger
Gloria Fernández-Esparrach
Moti Freiman
Weimin Huang

Xin Kang
Yogesh Karpate
David Kügler
Henry Krumb
Nerea Mangado
Awais Mansoor
Anirban Mukhopadhyay
Mauricio Reyes
Carles Sanchez
Stephan Zidowitz

Contents

CLIP 2019

UNSURE 2019: Uncertainty Quantification and Noise Modelling

Probabilistic Surface Reconstruction with Unknown Correspondence

Dennis Madsen$^{(\boxtimes)}$, Thomas Vetter, and Marcel Lüthi

Department of Mathematics and Computer Science, University of Basel,
Basel, Switzerland
{dennis.madsen,thomas.vetter,marcel.luethi}@unibas.ch

Abstract. We frequently encounter the need to reconstruct the full 3D surface from a given part of a bone in areas such as orthopaedics and surgical planning. Once we establish correspondence between the partial surface and a Statistical Shape Model (SSM), the problem has an appealing solution. The most likely reconstruction, as well as the full posterior distribution of all possible surface completions, can be obtained in closed form with an SSM. In this paper, we argue that assuming known correspondence is unjustified for long bones. We show that this can lead to reconstructions, which greatly underestimate the uncertainty. Even worse, the ground truth solution is often deemed very unlikely under the posterior. Our main contribution is a method which allows us to estimate the posterior distribution of surfaces given partial surface information without making any assumptions about the correspondence. To this end, we use the Metropolis-Hastings algorithm to sample reconstructions with unknown pose and correspondence from the posterior distribution. We introduce a projection-proposal to propose shape and pose updates to the Markov-Chain, which lets us explore the posterior distribution much more efficiently than a standard random-walk proposal. We use less than 1% of the samples needed by a random-walk to explore the posterior. We compare our method with the analytically computed posterior distribution, which assumes fixed correspondence. The comparison shows that our method leads to much more realistic posterior estimates when only small fragments of the bones are available.

Keywords: Statistical Shape Model · Posterior estimation · Surface prediction · Surface uncertainty · Metropolis-Hastings

1 Introduction

Surface reconstruction is encountered in many different areas. The reconstructed surface can be used to guide the design of patient-specific implants in the medical area, or estimate the sex and ethnicity of an individual in forensic investigations [10,11]. When only incomplete data is available, SSMs can be used to determine the most likely complete surface [2,12,13]. Nevertheless, the reconstruction becomes wrong and overconfident if correspondence cannot be obtained.

© Springer Nature Switzerland AG 2019
H. Greenspan et al. (Eds.): CLIP 2019/UNSURE 2019, LNCS 11840, pp. 3–11, 2019.
https://doi.org/10.1007/978-3-030-32689-0_1

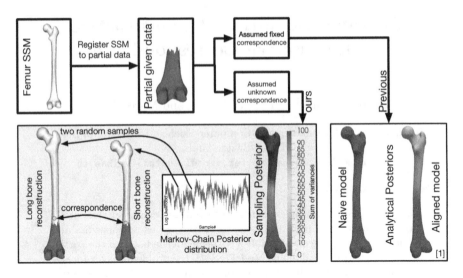

Fig. 1. A femur SSM is first registered to the partial surface to establish point-to-point correspondence. If we assume fixed correspondence, the posterior is computed analytically. With our method, we assume unknown correspondence and compute the posterior as a Markov-Chain. Note the correspondence difference to the available data visualised with the yellow markers on the long and short bone reconstructions. The coloured bones show the uncertainty, computed as the sum of the variances at each landmark with the different methods. Our method clearly shows more variability (red) far away from the partial surface, but at the same time has low variability (blue) at the known area. (Color figure online)

In cases where the surfaces are free of distinctive features, such as e.g. the shaft of a femur bone, there might even be multiple equally likely reconstructions with different lengths. In medical applications, a certainty estimate for a reconstruction is often required. This estimate can be computed as the likelihood of the chosen reconstruction in the distribution of all other possible reconstructions. Such a full distribution of surfaces given partial knowledge about the solution is known in the Bayesian setting as the posterior distribution. Since an SSM is formulated as a distribution over shapes, it is possible to derive a posterior model if only part of a surface is given [1] or if knowledge such as weight, sex, or age of a patient is known [3]. Current methods compute the posterior distribution analytically by assuming both fixed pose and fixed point-to-point correspondence [1,3]. Furthermore, the analytical-posterior requires an initial dataset alignment before it can be computed. In absence of exact point-to-point correspondence, those conditions are impossible to fulfil.

We present a method to estimate the posterior distribution from partial surface knowledge. A similar method has previously been used for fitting an active shape model to a target image [9] to compute the most likely solution. In contrast, we compute the full distribution of possible reconstructions.

In Fig. 1, we show how our method compares to the analytical method. We use the Metropolis-Hastings (MH) algorithm to compute the Markov-Chain posterior distribution. We will be referring to our method as the sampling-posterior.

The default random-walk in MH takes a long time to converge. As the SSM should stay fixed around the given part of the surface, we have to use very small shape and pose updates. Informed sampling approaches overcome this problem by including knowledge from the current state into its proposal [4, 7]. We introduce a new projection-proposal, which keeps the known part of the model fixed and only varies the pose and shape in the unknown part. In [8], an Iterative Closest Point (ICP)-like proposal is introduced for surface registration, whereas our projection-proposal explores the space of possible surface reconstructions of partial surfaces and includes the variability in pose difference.

We apply the sampling-posterior to estimate the posterior distribution of partial femurs. The femur bone is used as an example as the full shape of the femur (as well as other long bones) is inherently difficult to estimate. Thus, there is almost no correlation between the shape of the upper and lower part and the length. We show the limitations of the current method by comparing our sampling-posterior to the analytical-posterior distributions of different partial femur bones. This paper makes the following contributions:

- We show how to compute the estimated posterior distribution of a partial surface without assuming a fixed point-to-point correspondence in Sect. 3.1.
- We introduce a new MH proposal to create independent samples and thereby speed up the posterior estimation process in Sect. 3.2.
- We show the limitations of the current analytical-posterior [1] in Sect. 2.1 and based on experimental results in Sect. 4.

2 Statistical Shape Models

SSMs learn the shape variability from examples shapes. When working with a shape M_i, we usually work with the vector representation $s_i = (p^i_{1_x}, p^i_{1_y}, p^i_{1_z}, \ldots, p^i_{n_x}, p^i_{n_y}, p^i_{n_z})$ where $p \in \mathbb{R}^3$ is a landmark and n is the number of landmarks in the shape. A compact representation can be found by performing a Principal Component Analysis (PCA). The covariance matrix can then be represented by using $N - 1$ basis functions. In matrix format, the shapes are represented as $s = \mu + UD\alpha = \mu + Q\alpha$, with μ being the mean shape, U being the matrix containing all the eigenvectors and D containing the square-root of the eigenvalues of the covariance matrix Σ. Each shape M_i can then be determined by an α vector. The pose of the model can also be changed with both a translation vector $t = (t_x, t_y, t_z)^T \in \mathbb{R}^3$ and a rotation matrix parameterised by the Euler angles $R(\phi, \psi, \rho) \in SO(3)$. All parameters are concatenated into one vector $\theta = (\alpha_0, \ldots, \alpha_{N-1}, \phi, \psi, \rho, t_x, t_y, t_z)^T$ and we use the notation $M[\theta]$ to refer to the triangulated surface M defined by the parameter vector θ. The scale is directly incorporated in our construction of the SSM, as it would otherwise be difficult to obtain a correct statistical size measures if the size of the SSM can be scaled arbitrarily.

2.1 Analytical Posterior Models

We compare the sampling-posterior method to the analytical-posterior described in [1]. The given part of a shape is described as $s_g \in \mathbb{R}^{3q}$ with q being the number of landmarks. In our model, this becomes $s_g = \mu_g + Q_g\alpha + I_{3q}\epsilon$ with $\epsilon \sim \mathcal{N}(0, \sigma^2)$ being the noise term of each landmark observation. The difficulty with the analytical-posterior is that point-to-point correspondence needs to be obtained before the s_g vector can be defined. Furthermore, the rigid alignment needs to be fixed, resulting in the posterior distribution only containing shape variance.

In [1], the authors mention that all training shapes have to be aligned with respect to the subset of points available in s_g in order to have a meaningful result. In the following, we will refer to the analytical-posterior computed without aligning according to the s_g dataset as the naive-posterior and the analytical-posterior with the dataset alignment as the aligned-posterior.

3 Method

Now we explain how to compute the posterior distribution without assuming a fixed correspondence between the given data and the SSM. We define a probabilistic model over possible surface reconstructions (determined by θ) given partial surface information s_g,

$$P(\theta|s_g) = \frac{P(\theta)P(s_g|\theta)}{\int P(\theta)P(s_g|\theta)d\theta}. \tag{1}$$

The shape prior $P(\theta)$ penalises unlikely shapes. The combined likelihood over all the points in the given surface s_g is

$$P(s_g|\theta) = \prod_{i=1}^{q} \mathcal{N}(d_i(\theta, s_g); 0, \sigma^2), \tag{2}$$

where d_i is the Euclidean distance between the point p_i in the partial surface s_g to the closest point on the surface of $M[\theta]$. A similar likelihood function was used in [9] to measure the distance between an SSM and expert annotation in images. We define $\sigma^2 = 1.0\,\text{mm}^2$ and the same for ϵ in the analytical-posterior in order for the posterior distributions to be comparable. Note that the distance likelihood assumes that no pathologies exist in the partial surface.

3.1 Approximating the Probabilistic Model

Unfortunately, the full distribution of surfaces given the partial surface, as in Eq. (2), cannot be obtained analytically. Instead, it is possible to compute the unnormalised density for any surface described with θ. This allows us to use the MH algorithm to estimate the full posterior distribution. We use a random-walk to explore the shape space and have independent proposals for the translation $Q(t'|t)$, rotation $Q(R'|R)$, and shape $Q(\alpha'|\alpha)$ parameters. As scaling is directly incorporated in our SSM, a scaling proposal is not used.

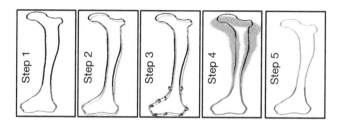

Fig. 2. Visualisation of the projection-proposal steps as described in Sect. 3.2. (Color figure online)

3.2 Projection-Proposal

Ideally, we would like to keep the known part of the shape model fixed around s_g, as we are interested in the posterior distribution given partial surface information. With the random-walk proposals, we have to use very small shape and pose update steps. As a consequence many samples need to be taken before independent samples are found. Therefore, we suggest a projection-proposal to keep the shape at the known part of the model fixed and only vary the unknown part. The projection-proposal makes use of the analytical-posterior as described in Sect. 2.1. Before computing the analytical-posterior, we make a random rotation or translation proposal and compute the posterior distribution based on the initial position of the model. When computing the analytical-posterior, an anisotropic noise term ϵ is used. To simulate correspondence shift along the surface, we model it as a multivariate normal distribution with a low variance along the normal and a higher variance along the surface. The variance at each point p_k in $M[\boldsymbol{\theta}]$ is computed by

$$\Sigma_{p_k} = [\boldsymbol{n}, \boldsymbol{v}_1, \boldsymbol{v}_2] \begin{bmatrix} \sigma_n^2 & 0 & 0 \\ 0 & \sigma_v^2 & 0 \\ 0 & 0 & \sigma_v^2 \end{bmatrix} [\boldsymbol{n}, \boldsymbol{v}_1, \boldsymbol{v}_2]^T \tag{3}$$

where $\boldsymbol{n}$ is the normal vector at the vertex $\boldsymbol{p}_k$ in the surface and $\boldsymbol{v}_1$ and $\boldsymbol{v}_2$ are perpendicular vectors to the normal. The variance along each vectors is set as $\sigma_n^2 = 0.1\,\text{mm}^2$ and $\sigma_v^2 = 5.0\,\text{mm}^2$. The projection-proposal can be described in 5 steps with Fig. 2 as visualisation for each step:

1. Compute corresponding points by taking the closest points from the partial surface (red) s_g to the current surface $M[\boldsymbol{\theta}]$ (black). We compute s_{g*} as the points in the SSM corresponding to the partial surface.
2. Propose a random pose update from $Q(t'|t) + Q(\boldsymbol{R'}|\boldsymbol{R})$, while keeping the current shape parameters $\boldsymbol{\alpha}$ fixed, such that a new $\boldsymbol{\theta}'$ is computed ($M[\boldsymbol{\theta}']$ shown in blue).
3. Compute the analytical-posterior $p(\boldsymbol{\alpha}|\boldsymbol{\theta}', s_{g*})$ based on Sect. 2.1.
4. Draw a sample from the distribution $p(\boldsymbol{\alpha}|\boldsymbol{\theta}', s_{g*})$ by randomly setting the $\boldsymbol{\alpha}$ vector in the SSM (green shows the posterior mean).

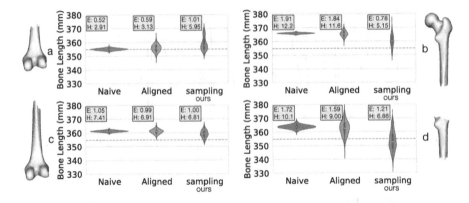

Fig. 3. Violin and box plots of bone length prediction in mm using the analytical-posterior and our sampling-posterior. All plots (a, b, c, d) concern the same ground-truth bone (length visualised with the red-dashed line), but differ in how much of the bone is given. The average Euclidean (E) and Hausdorff (H) distances from the ground-truth surface to the mean surface from the distributions are in mm. (Color figure online)

5. Compute the θ'' update based on the full SSM $p(\alpha)$ (the proposed sample $M[\theta'']$ is shown in green).

Unlike the random-walk proposal, this proposal is not symmetric. Therefore, to ensure convergence of the MH algorithm, we need to be able to compute the transition probabilities of going from θ to θ' as well as from θ' to θ [6]. The transition probability can be computed using the posterior distribution from step 3 as also shown in [8].

Projection-Proposal Importance. We need i.i.d. samples to compute the variance, which means that we need to find the number of samples to be discarded from the Markov-Chain before an independent sample is found. We compute the autocorrelation of the individual shape parameters and look for the number of samples needed to reach 0 correlation. We report 50 samples for the projection-proposal and 30×10^3 samples for the random-walk. While the random-walk requires 600 times more samples, the projection-proposal is only 6 times slower, making it overall 100 times faster.

We compute the bone length variance based on the distance between two landmarks. The length variation converges at 10^3 samples with the projection-proposal. For the random-walk, we need 500×10^3 samples to achieve the same length variance. With the projection-proposal, we can, therefore, explore similar variance numbers with less than 1% of the samples needed by the random-walk.

4   Evaluation

For the experiments, we use 61 femur meshes extracted from Computed Tomography (CT) images. We use 50 femurs for the femur SSM (femur lengths, mean:

372 mm, min: 322 mm, max: 437 mm) and 11 for the test-set (femur lengths, mean: 372 mm, min: 322 mm, max: 441 mm). The SSM contains a total of 1622 landmarks. Each test femur is divided into several partial meshes from where the posteriors are estimated. In Fig. 3, a subset of the cuts are shown[1].

Experimental Setup. We compare the sampling-posterior with the naive-posterior and the aligned-posterior. For the aligned-posterior, we need to estimate the observed points in the SSM. This is the same procedure that was done in step 1 of the projection-proposal. We perform a registration with the SSM and take the closest points to it from s_g. For the registration, we use the method from [9]. Alternatively, the non-rigid ICP algorithm can be used [5].

In the overview image of our method (Fig. 1), the posterior variability of the different methods is visualised with colours on the full femur bone. Very little variance is maintained in the naive-posterior, which highlights the importance of dataset alignment when computing the analytical-posterior. The sampling-posterior contains 2 to 3 times more variability than the aligned-posterior, suggesting that the full variability cannot be obtained using a fixed correspondence.

Length Estimation of Partial Bones. We compare the mean and the variance of bone lengths from the different posterior estimation methods. A landmark is placed at each end of the femur bones and the variability of the distance between the two landmarks is reported. For the analytical-posteriors, we randomly sample 10^3 shapes from the posterior models to be used for the estimate. For the projection-proposal we take 10^3 samples with 50 sample spacing in between. The bone length results for test femur 1 are shown in Fig. 3. Notice the difference between the results for partial bone a and c. More data is available in c, which results in a more narrow distribution, whereas the correspondence used in c is worse, making the ground-truth surface very unlikely under its distribution. The sampling-posterior results of the remaining test femurs are shown in Fig. 5.

We observe that both of the analytical-posterior methods sometimes fail to estimate the ground-truth length within their variability for most of the cuts. In contrast, the sampling-posterior can explain the shape length accurately.

Importance of Correct Correspondence. The quality of a surface reconstruction can be measured with the average Euclidean or Hausdorff distance to the ground-truth. These measures are, however, not a good indicator for the registration quality when large uncertainty exists in the correspondence. In Fig. 4 we show the same bone length experiment as in Fig. 3, but only for the aligned-posterior computed using different correspondences. The different correspondences have been found by initialising the SSM either as a very short, medium or long bone. We see that a close to perfect reconstruction can be found if the ground-truth correspondence is known, but at the same time can extremely over

---

[1] All experiments are performed with the open source-library https://scalismo.org.

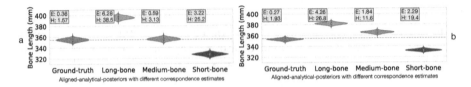

Fig. 4. Violin and box plots of bone length prediction in mm. All plots concern the same ground-truth bone (length visualised with the red-dashed line). The posteriors are computed with the aligned-analytical-posterior method and differ only in the correspondence which has been used. The average Euclidean (E) and Hausdorff (H) distances from the ground-truth surface to the mean surface from the distributions are in mm. (a) and (b) refers to the same partial shapes as in Fig. 3. (Color figure online)

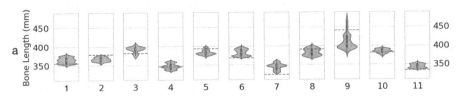

Fig. 5. Violin and box plots of bone length prediction in mm. All plots of different ground-truth bones. The posteriors are computed with our sampling method.

or underestimate the bone length if wrong correspondences is used. The average Euclidean distance from the partial surface to the reconstruction is, in all the cases, less than 0.25 mm, which suggests that the model represents the surface well in the available part.

5   Conclusion

It is difficult to infer the full shape from a bone fragment. This is due to missing exact point-to-point correspondence. Previous methods deterministically find a set of correspondences to estimate the posterior. This can results in overconfident posterior estimates if incorrect correspondences are used. We have shown how previous methods even fail to explain the ground truth solution in an experimental setup with synthetic data. Our main contribution is a sampling approach that estimates the posterior distribution without relying on a fixed set of correspondences. We use the MH algorithm to obtain the variability in shape and pose reconstruction of partial surfaces. We have shown that the sampling-posterior, in contrast to the analytical methods, robustly is able to explain ground-truth data under its posterior. We also presented a technical contribution to the sampling-posterior in the form of a projection-proposal. This proposal is able to explore the posterior distribution more efficiently. With our sampling-posterior approach, both correspondence and reconstruction estimates are more accurate than with the traditional analytical approach. We are also able to more reliably estimate the uncertainty of the reconstruction results.

Acknowledgements. This research is sponsored by the Gebert Rüf Foundation under the project GRS-029/17.

References

1. Albrecht, T., Lüthi, M., Gerig, T., Vetter, T.: Posterior shape models. Med. Image Anal. **17**(8), 959–973 (2013)
2. Bernard, F., et al.: Shape-aware surface reconstruction from sparse 3D point-clouds. Med. Image Anal. **38**, 77–89 (2017)
3. Blanc, R., Reyes, M., Seiler, C., Székely, G.: Conditional variability of statistical shape models based on surrogate variables. In: Yang, G.-Z., Hawkes, D., Rueckert, D., Noble, A., Taylor, C. (eds.) MICCAI 2009. LNCS, vol. 5762, pp. 84–91. Springer, Heidelberg (2009). https://doi.org/10.1007/978-3-642-04271-3_11
4. Cui, T., Law, K.J., Marzouk, Y.M.: Dimension-independent likelihood-informed mcmc. J. Comput. Phys. **304**, 109–137 (2016)
5. Feldmar, J., Ayache, N.: Rigid, affine and locally affine registration of free-form surfaces. Int. J. Comput. Vision **18**(2), 99–119 (1996)
6. Hastings, W.K.: Monte Carlo sampling methods using Markov chains and their applications (1970)
7. Kortylewski, A., et al.: Informed MCMC with Bayesian neural networks for facial image analysis. arXiv preprint arXiv:1811.07969 (2018)
8. Madsen, D., Morel-Forster, A., Kahr, P., Rahbani, D., Vetter, T., Lüthi, M.: A closest point proposal for MCMC-based probabilistic surface registration. arXiv preprint arXiv:1907.01414 (2019)
9. Morel-Forster, A., Gerig, T., Lüthi, M., Vetter, T.: Probabilistic fitting of active shape models. In: Reuter, M., Wachinger, C., Lombaert, H., Paniagua, B., Lüthi, M., Egger, B. (eds.) ShapeMI 2018. LNCS, vol. 11167, pp. 137–146. Springer, Cham (2018). https://doi.org/10.1007/978-3-030-04747-4_13
10. Purkait, R.: Triangle identified at the proximal end of femur: a new sex determinant. Forensic Sci. Int. **147**(2–3), 135–139 (2005)
11. Trotter, M., Gleser, G.C.: Estimation of stature from long bones of american whites and negroes. Am. J. Phys. Anthropol. **10**(4), 463–514 (1952)
12. Zheng, G., et al.: Accurate and robust reconstruction of a surface model of the proximal femur from sparse-point data and a dense-point distribution model for surgical navigation. IEEE Trans. Biomed. Eng. **54**(12), 2109–2122 (2007)
13. Zhu, Z., Li, G.: Construction of 3D human distal femoral surface models using a 3D statistical deformable model. J. Biomech. **44**(13), 2362–2368 (2011)

Probabilistic Image Registration via Deep Multi-class Classification: Characterizing Uncertainty

Alireza Sedghi[1]([✉]), Tina Kapur[2], Jie Luo[2,3], Parvin Mousavi[1], and William M. Wells III[2]

[1] Medical Informatics Laboratory, Queen's University, Kingston, ON, Canada
sedghi@cs.queensu.ca
[2] Radiology Department, Brigham and Women's Hospital, Harvard Medical School, Boston, MA, USA
[3] Graduate School of Frontier Sciences, The University of Tokyo, Tokyo, Japan

Abstract. We present a novel approach to probabilistic image registration that leverages the strengths of deep-learning for modeling agreement between images. We use a deep multi-class classifier trained on different classes of patch pairs, including *unrelated, registered,* and a collection of discrete displacements between patches. The displacement classes alleviate the need for registration-time optimization by gradient descent; instead, posterior probabilities are used to directly predict expected values of displacements on the lattice of sampled locations. These, in turn, are used to update transformation parameters and the process is iterated. We empirically demonstrate the accuracy of our proposed method on deformable cross-modality registrations of brain MRI, and show improved results compared to Mutual Information based method on challenging data that includes simulated resections. Our approach enables local predictions of registration uncertainty and diagnostics that can indicate areas that seem unrelated in the two images. Uncertainty estimates provide end-users with intuitively actionable information on the quality of registration in interventional and surgical settings.

1 Introduction

Image registration is a critical element in many image-guided therapy applications. For instance, commercially available neuro-navigation systems that register pre-operative images to the intra-operative coordinate space of the patient are used routinely by neurosurgeons to perform brain tumor resection [5,15]. A highly desirable feature of such systems would be to use non-rigid registration methods to incorporate intra-operatively acquired images that show changes due to brain shift and tumor resection. Given that currently available non-rigid registration methods do not lead to perfect results for such tasks, it would be very beneficial for the registration systems to also predict local estimates of the registration uncertainty. This information could be used to alert the user to not

© Springer Nature Switzerland AG 2019
H. Greenspan et al. (Eds.): CLIP 2019/UNSURE 2019, LNCS 11840, pp. 12–22, 2019.
https://doi.org/10.1007/978-3-030-32689-0_2

depend critically on the registration results if the predicted uncertainty is too high. Also, users may be more willing to use such systems if they have confidence in the registration results when the system predicts low uncertainty, in comparison to imperfect registration systems that do not report uncertainty.

Related Work. Prior to the emergence of deep learning-based registration methods, continuous [13,16,21,25] or discrete [6–8,24] probabilistic registration approaches were used to characterize uncertainty in registration results. For instance, Glocker *et al.* [6] describe a discrete formulation of non-rigid registration that can be used with any agreement measure. The system iterates updates on control points that are solved by linear programming. A subsequent probabilistic formulation [7] estimates min-marginal distributions that characterize local uncertainty in the result. Most deep learning registration methods model the transformation parameters in a non-probabilistic fashion [4,12,18,22,23]. A few recent deep learning approaches have incorporated uncertainty estimates of registration. Balakrishnan *et al.* [1] proposed VoxelMorph, an unsupervised learning approach where a deep network is trained to minimize a conventional dissimilarity measure (i.e., mean squared intensity difference) between the images. Later, they extended their framework in [3] to generate registration uncertainty. Yang *et al.* [26] proposed a deep encoder-decoder regression model to predict the momentum parameterization for diffeomorphic registration. They utilize Bayesian dropout layers in their network which enables estimation of the uncertainty by sampling multiple momentum predictions from the network.

Discriminative methods for image registration have been introduced that learn to classify patches of images based on deep learning. Simonovsky *et al.* [20] proposed Deep Metric Registration (DMR) that uses class-labeled data to train a deep binary classifier and use it as an effective similarity metrics for pairwise multi-modal image registration. The essential idea in the DMR approach is to prepare two classes of training data. One class, referred to as *registered*, contains pairs of corresponding patches, while the other, referred to as *unrelated*, contains pairs of patches that are randomly and independently sampled in location. The class-labeled patch pairs are used to train a deep classifier (semi-supervised methods have also been investigated to train such a deep metric classifier in [19]). Subsequently, at registration time, the posterior probability that patches are registered is used as a measure of image agreement, and an aggregate score over a collection of patch pairs is optimized through gradient descent.

Contributions. In this paper we present a novel formulation of deep classifier-based image registration that goes beyond binary classification. In addition to the *unrelated* and *registered* classes, we include classes corresponding to a collection of discrete displacements. Including the displacement classes alleviates the need for registration-time optimization by gradient descent; instead, posterior probabilities on classes are used to directly predict expected values of displacements on the lattice of sampled locations. These, in turn, are used to update transformation parameters and the process is iterated. We empirically demonstrate that the iteration exhibits steady convergence. Our approach has similarities to Glocker's probabilistic variant of discrete non-rigid registration [7].

Differences include (1) while both predict posterior distributions on displacement, we include an *unrelated* class that can be used to explain image areas that do not seem to agree, (2) we use deep learning classifiers to predict displacements, (3) our updates are based on very simple and inexpensive calculations on classifier results rather than linear programming and min-marginal calculations. To the best of our knowledge, this is the first registration method that uses deep networks to learn image agreement and that produces estimates of registration uncertainty along with the probability that the image contents are unrelated.

The paper is organized as follows. In Sect. 2 we describe our multi-class classifier training and the registration algorithm. In Sect. 3 we investigate the performance of our proposed method and compare it with the widely used Elastix registration package [11] on multiple experiments. Finally, we compare our uncertainty prediction to the actual error of registration.

2   Methods

We use probabilistic predictions from a CNN-based multi-class classifier to drive image registration. The final predictions are used to estimate the local uncertainty (variance) in the displacements, as well as to indicate that the images may include different contents, locally.

Classification-Network: We define 20 classes of patch pairs, $c_{i=1}^{20}$, including *unrelated, registered,* and 18 classes that correspond to $\pm2, \pm4, \pm8$ voxel displacements in the $x, y,$ and z directions between the two patches. We also define $d_{i=3}^{20}$ as the displacements (mm) associated with $c_{i=3}^{20}$, and we set d_1 and d_2 (corresponding to *unrelated* and *registered* classes) to zero displacements. The classifier design is inspired by densely connected networks [9] with 3D convolutions. Early fusion of the information between two images has shown to be superior to the other methods for patch comparison [27]; therefore, we use two-channel input where 3D patch pairs from the fixed and moving images are concatenated. The network has 20 outputs corresponding to the probabilities of an input patch pair belonging to class c_i. We train our CNN by minimizing the cross-entropy loss between the true class labels $y \in c_i$ and the predicted class probabilities.

Image Registration: After training the classifier, registration proceeds as:
Initialize a rectangular grid of control points that cover the moving image. For B-spline registration these will serve as the transformation parameters; for affine or rigid registration initialize the respective transformation parameters.
Iterate (1) Transform the moving image according to current transformation parameters. (2) Extract 3D patches from the transformed moving image and the corresponding locations in the fixed image that are centered on the control points. (3) Run the classifier on the patch pairs, obtaining class probabilities, and calculate, for each pair, the expected displacement, variance, and probability of being unrelated. (4) For B-spline models, increment the control points with their respective expected displacements; otherwise, use the control points and predicted displacements to calculate a least squares estimate of the rigid/affine transformation parameters.

For N cropped pairs of patches, we calculate expected displacements (D) as: $D = [\mathbb{E}_{y_1}[d] \; \mathbb{E}_{y_2}[d] \; ... \; \mathbb{E}_{y_N}[d]]$ where $\mathbb{E}_{y_j}[d] = \sum_{i=1}^{20} p(y_j = c_i)d_i$. Here, $p(y_j = c_i)$ is the posterior probability of the jth input patch pair belonging to class c_i, and d_i is the associated displacement. The probability that the jth patch pair is *unrelated*, $p(y_j = c_1)$, infers that images do not contain related content, locally. Our proposed approach takes advantage of this information by explicitly setting d_1, the displacement of the *unrelated* class, to zero. As a result, image patches that have little related content will not have much effect on displacements. We hypothesize that modeling the *unrelated* class increases the robustness of the registration system, which is borne out in the experiments below. In future work, we will investigate assigning the value of a spatial regularizer for the displacement associated with the *unrelated* class.

Uncertainty Estimation: As stated before, registration uncertainty plays a potentially critical role in assessing the utility of image registration. In contrast to conventional regression approaches, we can easily calculate posterior uncertainty, so at the final location of the control points, we calculate a scalar variance as $\sigma_j^2 = \mathbb{E}_{y_j}\left[|d - \mathbb{E}_{y_j}[d]|^2\right]$, along with $u_j = p(y_j = c_1)$. Both variance and *the probability of being unrelated* are interpolated using a Radial Basis Function (RBF) spline covering the image space.

3 Experiments and Results

Data: We carry out experiments using the IXI dataset [10] which contains multiple-sequences of aligned brain MRI images of healthy subjects. These include T1 and T2 weighted MRI. We also include synthetic Gradient Magnitude (GradMag) images that we compute from T2. We use non-overlapping sets of 50 subjects for training the CNN classifier, 15 for validation, and 50 for testing and reporting the registration performance. All images are initially re-aligned (within subjects) to compensate for possible residual misregistrations, and resampled to a $1 \times 1 \times 1$ mm. For each class of displaced patch pairs, $c_{i=3}^{20}$, we translate the moving image according to its class displacement, d_i before cropping. For *unrelated* class, we crop patches from different random locations in the fixed and moving images. Overall, 60,000 patch pairs of voxel-size $17 \times 17 \times 17$ are generated for each class, which results in 1.2 million patch pairs for training.

Training: Our 3D densenet classifier architecture consists of 4 dense blocks with 10 initial filters and growth rates of 16. During training, the Adam update rule with an initial learning rate of 10^{-4}, batch size of 256 and ℓ_2-regularization of $5e^{-4}$ is used to optimize the network. All the hyperparameters (both architecture and training parameters) are empirically estimated to achieve maximum accuracy in the validation data.

Baseline: Our baseline is the well-known publicly available Elastix [11] registration package. Elastix parameters ("number of samples": 2048, "metric": "Normalized Mutual Information (NMI)" or "Cross-correlation (NCC)", "optimizer": "Adaptive SGD", "number of iterations": 512,) are validated to be optimum.

We perform rigid, affine and deformable registration experiments to assess the performance of our proposed method and to quantify the relationship of our predicted uncertainty to the actual error of registration. For rigid/affine experiments, we apply random initial transformations to misregister the images and find the transformation that aligns them. We report Fiducial Registration Error (FRE), calculated from 100 arbitrary sparse landmarks, from their initial positions and those following final registration. For the deformable experiments, we use overlap scores (mean Dice) as measures of agreement [2] between grey matter (GM), white matter (WM), and cerebrospinal fluid (CSF), computed by FSL FAST algorithm [28]. Finally, we compare our uncertainty estimates to the actual error of registration in the deformable registration experiments and plot them together. Average running time of our method is 0.32 ± 0.1 and 0.59 ± 0.08 seconds per iteration for rigid/affine and B-spline registration respectively using GeForce GTX 1080 Ti which puts runtime of our iterated approach within clinically acceptable margins for neurosurgery [17].

3.1   Rigid Registration and Parameter Update Range

To explore the parameter update range of our method, we train a classifier on T1 and T2-weighted patches with 20 classes of displacements. Next, for a random fixed image (T2) in the test set, the corresponding moving image (T1) is translated in x, y, z directions by different values (from $-8\,\mathrm{mm}$ to $8\,\mathrm{mm}$, with $0.5\,\mathrm{mm}$ steps). For each translation experiment, we calculate the expected value of displacements for 100 randomly cropped patches ($\mathbb{E}_{y_j}[d]\ j = 1, ..., 100$). Finally, we plot the average predicted displacement for each translation experiment in Fig. 1(a). It is clear that our model, while trained on discrete displacements, can correctly predict a close approximation of the actual displacement (almost linear trend); thus, it can make rapid progress to convergence.

Our method can be easily adapted for a multi-resolution registration schema. We demonstrate this using a test case with 5 different scales of initial error (FRE of 5, 10, 20, 40, 60 mm). Three different classifiers are trained on 3 resolutions of the data (Model1 on 1 mm voxel spacings, Model2 on 2 mm, and Model3 on 3 mm) for the $c_{i=1}^{20}$. Class definitions remain the same at all scales. We use Model3, Model2, and Model1 to capture large, medium and small misalignments respectively. The convergence plot for the models is depicted in Fig. 1(b). We observe that large initial misalignments can be easily compensated by Model3 (purple) while the model at the finest scale can give the best accuracy (blue). Therefore, a multi-resolution pyramid registration approach can be built using the proposed method in which we use coarser models to start the optimization and switch to finer scale models after.

A natural question is whether or not a registration method that has a CNN classifier trained on translated images can perform well on rotated images. To address this, we perform multiple rigid registrations for T2 and rotated T1 (0.1–0.8 rad) of a test subject and plot the convergence during registration. As seen in Fig. 1(c) we are able to achieve voxel-level FRE even with initial rotations of 0.8 rad (nearly $45°$).

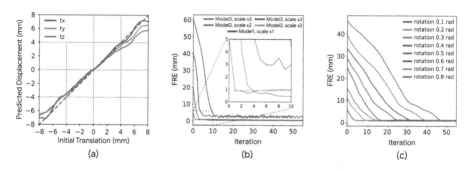

Fig. 1. (a) Predicted displacement in mm in *y-axis*, and initial translation in mm in *x-axis*. (b) Convergence plot for small and big initial misregistrations using 3 models trained on different resolution. (c) Convergence plot of rigid registration based on different amount of rotational misalignment. (Color figure online)

3.2 Affine Multi-modality Registration

We generate GradMag images for 3D MRI volumes, and perform affine registration of these to T2 images. GradMag images have contrast somewhat similar to ultrasound, mimicking a multi-modality registration problem. After training a CNN classifier for T2 and GradMag patches (the same hyperparameters were used for the architecture and training), we substantially misalign the moving images with 100 different affine transformations and try to register them back. The Affine parameters are sampled from $\mathcal{U}_t\{1, 25\}$, $\mathcal{U}_\theta\{0.01, 0.2\}$, $\mathcal{U}_s\{0.95, 1.05\}$ and $\mathcal{U}_{sh}\{-0.05, 0.05\}$ for translation, rotation, scale and shear, respectively. This led to an initial error of 20.69 ± 4.88 mm in the test set. The trained CNN is used to register the data as described in Sect. 2. We achieved final FRE of 0.82 ± 0.44 mm, substantially outperforming Elastix, which achieved final FRE of 4.61 ± 2.50 mm and 2.71 ± 1.20 mm respectively for normalized mutual information and normalized cross-correlation metrics.

3.3 Deformable Registration and Uncertainty Estimation

Inter-subject registration is challenging as some cortical structures may exist in only the moving or the fixed image. Our first experiment involves 100 inter-subject multi-resolution (2 scales) B-spline registrations. In this preliminary experiment, we use a relatively coarse grid of $10 \times 10 \times 10$ at the finest level. For each registration experiment, we randomly select two images from our test set (T2 from one subject, and T1 from a different subject) and register them using our trained classifier, as explained before.

Registration of pre- and intra-operative images is a desired feature in image-guided surgery, and it could have the most utility after resection has been carried out. Unfortunately, resection makes the registration problem more difficult. To simulate this scenario, we created another test dataset by putting synthesized resected areas, in different sizes and shapes, in random locations of the

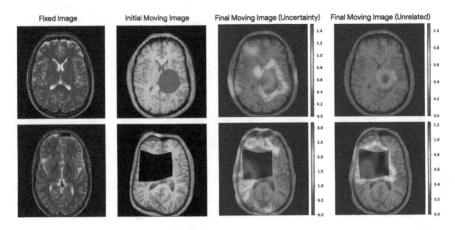

Fig. 2. Intra-subject deformable registration and results. The first column of each row is a pre-operative T2 MRI axial cross-section, the second column is a simulated post-resection image created by blanking out a region of T1 MRI, the third column is our registered T1 MRI (moving image) overlaid with uncertainty values, and the fourth column is the registered T1 MRI (moving image) overlaid with *probability of being unrelated*. In the third and fourth columns, Red indicates higher standard deviation and higher probability of *unrelated* class, respectively. (Color figure online)

T1 images (see Fig. 2). We perform 200 intra-subject multi-resolution (2 scales) B-spline registrations of T2 and T1-resected images. For each experiment, we randomly perturb the control points of the B-spline grid (on the moving image) with displacements following a uniform distribution $\mathcal{U}\{-25, 25\}$ mm, and we try to register the images back to their initial configuration. We also perform an experiment by using a CNN classifier that is not trained on the *unrelated* class data (only trained to distinguish 18 class of displacements and the *registered* class).

The results of both experiments are reported in Table 1. As seen, for the inter-subject experiment, our method achieves accuracies comparable to Elastix,

Table 1. Mean Dice score of GM, WM, and CSF for inter- and intra subject deformable registration of T1 and T2 with Elastix and our proposed method. "*" indicates statistically significant difference between results (t-test, $p < 0.001$).

	Dice score, inter-subj			Dice score, intra-subj + "resection"		
	GM	WM	CSF	GM	WM	CSF
Initial	0.36 ± 0.07	0.45 ± 0.09	0.18 ± 0.06	0.47 ± 0.05	0.57 ± 0.04	0.30 ± 0.05
Elastix	0.48 ± 0.04	$0.66 \pm 0.02^*$	0.32 ± 0.03	0.67 ± 0.04	0.77 ± 0.04	0.55 ± 0.06
Proposed	$0.52 \pm 0.02^*$	0.64 ± 0.01	$0.35 \pm 0.03^*$	$0.70 \pm 0.03^*$	0.77 ± 0.03	$0.62 \pm 0.04^*$
Proposed	(w/o *unrelated class*)			0.49 ± 0.05	0.63 ± 0.06	0.34 ± 0.07

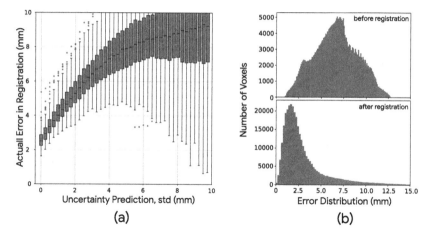

Fig. 3. Distribution of error and uncertainty for intra-subject registration experiment. (a) error distribution for different discretized uncertainty intervals (first interval $0 < u \leq 0.25$ and so on) (b) distribution of error before and after registration for a test case.

and for the more challenging experiment with the virtual resected regions, our performance is significantly higher.

At the final location of the control points we calculate the scalar standard deviation of the displacements as the estimated uncertainty and also $p(y_j = c_1)$ which represents the probability that patches are *unrelated*, and interpolate them to cover image space. We depict these predictive diagnostics for two intra-subject deformable registrations in Fig. 2. As seen, our model has detected the areas that have *unrelated* contents (resected regions), and surrounding areas have higher uncertainty (standard deviation) as expected. We suspect the lack of correspondence between the pre- and intra-operative images is the reason for the large uncertainty at the resected area.

3.4 Evaluation of Uncertainty Estimates

As the ground-truth of the intra-subject experiment is known, we investigate the relationship between the predicted uncertainty (standard deviation) and the actual registration error [14]. The result of this analysis for the population of 200 registration experiments is shown in Fig. 3. In Fig. 3(a) each bar plot presents a summary of registration error and predicted uncertainty over a population of subjects. We have discretized the uncertainty prediction into 0.25 mm intervals for ease of visualization. We observe a strong positive linear relationship between the uncertainty and actual errors of registration ($r = 0.94$ with $p < 0.001$), and importantly, low levels of predicted uncertainty correspond to low levels of actual error.

4   Conclusions and Future Work

We presented an efficient and flexible approach based on deep multi-class classifiers for multimodal 3D image registration that predicts estimated displacements of pairs of patches. Our method does not need any optimization on the transformation parameters as it uses a sequence of approximate solutions that empirically exhibit good convergence. The experimental evaluation of rigid, affine and deformable image registration demonstrates the effectiveness of our method. Our method achieved statistically significant improvements in performance compared to the widely-used image registration toolkit Elastix. We were able to directly quantify the uncertainty of the registration with our probabilistic classifier, and show that our predicted uncertainty is strongly predictive of actual errors. This information could be valuable in decision making for interventional applications.

For future work, we will pursue registration of pre-operative MRI to intra-operative MRI as well as to ultrasound, where conventional metrics have difficulties. In addition, we will extend our methodology to operate on the whole image instead of only the control points and compare our method to other discrete approaches.

Acknowledgements. Research reported in this publication was supported by Natural Sciences and Engineering Research Council (NSERC) of Canada, the Canadian Institutes of Health Research (CIHR), Ontario Trillium Scholarship, NIH Grant P41EB015898.

References

1. Balakrishnan, G., Zhao, A., Sabuncu, M.R., Guttag, J., Dalca, A.V.: An unsupervised learning model for deformable medical image registration. In: Proceedings of the IEEE CVPR, pp. 9252–9260 (2018)
2. Cao, X., et al.: Deformable image registration based on similarity-steered CNN regression. In: Descoteaux, M., Maier-Hein, L., Franz, A., Jannin, P., Collins, D.L., Duchesne, S. (eds.) MICCAI 2017. LNCS, vol. 10433, pp. 300–308. Springer, Cham (2017). https://doi.org/10.1007/978-3-319-66182-7_35
3. Dalca, A.V., Balakrishnan, G., Guttag, J., Sabuncu, M.R.: Unsupervised learning for fast probabilistic diffeomorphic registration. In: Frangi, A.F., Schnabel, J.A., Davatzikos, C., Alberola-López, C., Fichtinger, G. (eds.) MICCAI 2018. LNCS, vol. 11070, pp. 729–738. Springer, Cham (2018). https://doi.org/10.1007/978-3-030-00928-1_82
4. Fan, J., Cao, X., Yap, P., Shen, D.: BIRNet: brain image registration using dual-supervised fully convolutional networks. Med. Image Anal. 128–143 (2019)
5. Gerard, I., Kersten-Oertel, M., Petrecca, K., Sirhan, D., Hall, J., Collins, D.: Brain shift in neuronavigation of brain tumors: a review. Med. Image Anal. **35**, 403–420 (2017)
6. Glocker, B., Komodakis, N., Tziritas, G., Navab, N., Paragios, N.: Dense image registration through MRFs and efficient linear programming. Med. Image Anal. **12**(6), 731–741 (2008)

7. Glocker, B., Paragios, N., Komodakis, N., Tziritas, G., Navab, N.: Optical flow estimation with uncertainties through dynamic MRFs. In: IEEE CVPR, pp. 1–8 (2008)
8. Heinrich, M., Simpson, I., Papież, B., Brady, M., Schnabel, J.: Deformable image registration by combining uncertainty estimates from supervoxel belief propagation. Med. Image Anal. **27**, 57–71 (2016)
9. Huang, G., Liu, Z., Van Der Maaten, L., Weinberger, K.Q.: Densely connected convolutional networks. In: Proceedings of the IEEE CVPR, pp. 4700–4708 (2017)
10. IXI: Information eXtraction from Images. http://brain-development.org/
11. Klein, S., Staring, M., Murphy, K., Viergever, M.A., Pluim, J.P.: Elastix: a toolbox for intensity-based medical image registration. IEEE TMI **29**(1), 196–205 (2010)
12. Krebs, J., et al.: Robust non-rigid registration through agent-based action learning. In: Descoteaux, M., Maier-Hein, L., Franz, A., Jannin, P., Collins, D.L., Duchesne, S. (eds.) MICCAI 2017. LNCS, vol. 10433, pp. 344–352. Springer, Cham (2017). https://doi.org/10.1007/978-3-319-66182-7_40
13. Le Folgoc, L., Delingette, H., Criminisi, A., Ayache, N.: Quantifying registration uncertainty with sparse bayesian modelling. IEEE TMI **36**(2), 607–617 (2016)
14. Luo, J., Golby, A., Sugiyama, M., Wells III, W., Frisken, S.: Pilot study on verifying the monotonic relationship between error and uncertainty in deformable registration for neurosurgery. arXiv:1908.07709v1
15. Luo, J., et al.: A feature-driven active framework for ultrasound-based brain shift compensation. In: Frangi, A.F., Schnabel, J.A., Davatzikos, C., Alberola-López, C., Fichtinger, G. (eds.) MICCAI 2018. LNCS, vol. 11073, pp. 30–38. Springer, Cham (2018). https://doi.org/10.1007/978-3-030-00937-3_4
16. Risholm, P., Janoos, F., Norton, I., Golby, A., Wells, W.M.: Bayesian characterization of uncertainty in intra-subject non-rigid registration. Med. Image Anal. **17**, 538–555 (2013)
17. Risholm, P., Golby, A.J., Wells, W.M.: Multimodal image registration for preoperative planning and image-guided neurosurgical procedures. Neurosurg. Clin. **22**(2), 197–206 (2011)
18. Rohé, M.-M., Datar, M., Heimann, T., Sermesant, M., Pennec, X.: SVF-Net: learning deformable image registration using shape matching. In: Descoteaux, M., Maier-Hein, L., Franz, A., Jannin, P., Collins, D.L., Duchesne, S. (eds.) MICCAI 2017. LNCS, vol. 10433, pp. 266–274. Springer, Cham (2017). https://doi.org/10.1007/978-3-319-66182-7_31
19. Sedghi, A., et al.: Semi-supervised image registration using deep learning. In: Proceedings of SPIE the International Society for Optical Engineering, vol. 10951, p. 109511G (2019)
20. Simonovsky, M., Gutiérrez-Becker, B., Mateus, D., Navab, N., Komodakis, N.: A deep metric for multimodal registration. In: Ourselin, S., Joskowicz, L., Sabuncu, M.R., Unal, G., Wells, W. (eds.) MICCAI 2016. LNCS, vol. 9902, pp. 10–18. Springer, Cham (2016). https://doi.org/10.1007/978-3-319-46726-9_2
21. Simpson, I.J., Schnabel, J.A., Groves, A.R., Andersson, J.L., Woolrich, M.W.: Probabilistic inference of regularisation in non-rigid registration. NeuroImage **59**(3), 2438–2451 (2012)
22. Sokooti, H., de Vos, B., Berendsen, F., Lelieveldt, B.P.F., Išgum, I., Staring, M.: Nonrigid image registration using multi-scale 3D convolutional neural networks. In: Descoteaux, M., Maier-Hein, L., Franz, A., Jannin, P., Collins, D.L., Duchesne, S. (eds.) MICCAI 2017. LNCS, vol. 10433, pp. 232–239. Springer, Cham (2017). https://doi.org/10.1007/978-3-319-66182-7_27

23. de Vos, B., Berendsen, F., Viergever, M., Sokooti, H., Staring, M., Isgum, I.: A deep learning framework for unsupervised affine and deformable image registration. Med. Image Anal. **52**, 128–143 (2019)

24. Popuri, K., Cobzas, D., Jägersand, M.: A variational formulation for discrete registration. In: Mori, K., Sakuma, I., Sato, Y., Barillot, C., Navab, N. (eds.) MICCAI 2013. LNCS, vol. 8151, pp. 187–194. Springer, Heidelberg (2013). https://doi.org/10.1007/978-3-642-40760-4_24

25. Wang, J., Wells, W.M., Golland, P., Zhang, M.: Efficient laplace approximation for bayesian registration uncertainty quantification. In: Frangi, A.F., Schnabel, J.A., Davatzikos, C., Alberola-López, C., Fichtinger, G. (eds.) MICCAI 2018. LNCS, vol. 11070, pp. 880–888. Springer, Cham (2018). https://doi.org/10.1007/978-3-030-00928-1_99

26. Yang, X., Kwitt, R., Styner, M., Niethammer, M.: Quicksilver: fast predictive image registration-a deep learning approach. NeuroImage **158**, 378–396 (2017)

27. Zagoruyko, S., Komodakis, N.: Learning to compare image patches via convolutional neural networks. In: Proceedings of the IEEE CVPR, pp. 4353–4361 (2015)

28. Zhang, Y., Brady, M., Smith, S.: Segmentation of brain mr images through a hidden markov random field model and the expectation-maximization algorithm. IEEE TMI **20**(1), 45–57 (2001)

Propagating Uncertainty Across Cascaded Medical Imaging Tasks for Improved Deep Learning Inference

Raghav Mehta[1]([envelope]), Thomas Christinck[1], Tanya Nair[1], Paul Lemaitre[1], Douglas Arnold[2,3], and Tal Arbel[1]

[1] Centre for Intelligent Machines, McGill University, Montreal, Canada
raghav@cim.mcgill.ca
[2] Montreal Neurological Institute, McGill University, Montreal, Canada
[3] NeuroRx Research, Montreal, Canada

Abstract. Although deep networks have been shown to perform very well on a variety of tasks, inference in the presence of pathology in medical images presents challenges to traditional networks. Given that medical image analysis typically requires a sequence of inference tasks to be performed (e.g. registration, segmentation), this results in an accumulation of errors over the sequence of deterministic outputs. In this paper, we explore the premise that, by embedding uncertainty estimates across cascaded inference tasks, the final prediction results should improve over simply cascading the deterministic classification results or performing inference in a single stage. Specifically, we develop a deep learning framework that propagates voxel-based uncertainty measures (e.g. Monte Carlo (MC) dropout sample variance) across inference tasks in order to improve the detection and segmentation of focal pathologies (e.g. lesions, tumours) in brain MR images. We apply the framework to two different contexts. First, we demonstrate that propagating multiple sclerosis T2 lesion segmentation results along with their associated uncertainty measures improves subsequent T2 lesion detection accuracy when evaluated on a proprietary large-scale, multi-site, clinical trial dataset. Second, we show how by propagating uncertainties associated with a regressed 3D MRI volume as an additional input to a follow-on brain tumour segmentation task, one can improve segmentation results on the publicly available BraTS-2018 dataset.

1 Introduction

Deep learning methods have been shown to outperform other methods on a variety of medical imaging inference tasks [1–6]. However, challenges still remain in applying traditional networks to clinical tasks in the presence of focal pathologies. Given that a typical medical image analysis pipeline generally requires a sequence of inference tasks to be performed (e.g. registration, segmentation),

---

R. Mehta and T. Christinck—Equal contribution.

© Springer Nature Switzerland AG 2019
H. Greenspan et al. (Eds.): CLIP 2019/UNSURE 2019, LNCS 11840, pp. 23–32, 2019.
https://doi.org/10.1007/978-3-030-32689-0_3

errors made over the sequence of deterministic models can accumulate and affect the downstream clinical task of interest (e.g. survival prediction). For example, the reported underperformance of the popular U-Net in the detection and segmentation of very small lesions [5] is problematic in the context of Multiple Sclerosis (MS), in that detecting all lesions, including small ones, in patient MRI is important for disease staging, prognosis, and monitoring treatment efficacy. Recently, it has been shown that popular deep networks adapted for the synthesis of missing MRI sequences (e.g. FLAIR) underperform in the presence of tumours. This negatively affects the downstream tasks of tumour classification, and staging and sub-type segmentation [2,11] that rely on the presence of these sequences. In this paper, we hypothesize that the performance of the downstream tasks in a medical image analysis pipeline should improve if, in addition to deterministic predictions, uncertainty estimates are propagated across cascaded inference tasks.

Recently, Bayesian machine learning approaches have begun to address the limitation of deterministic deep learning methods by providing an uncertainty associated with each prediction. Gal and Ghahramani [7] showed that by training a neural network with dropout and taking Monte Carlo (MC) samples of the prediction using dropout at test time, one can estimate the uncertainty associated with the output of deep learning methods. MC dropout based uncertainty estimation has been used in a variety of medical imaging tasks recently [8–10], ranging from modality synthesis [2] to nodule detection [8] and lesion detection and segmentation [5]. Many of these papers report that prediction uncertainty can be used to estimate regions of an image where the network is prone to error [2,9]. Others demonstrate an improved performance when the network output is evaluated on its most certain predictions [5,10]. While these approaches illustrate how estimating uncertainty in medical imaging tasks is useful in a clinical scenario, they do not show how uncertainty can be used to inform or improve network performance on a downstream task. In [8], the authors begin to address this limitation by showing how uncertainty from a 2D lung nodule segmentation network can be used to reduce the *false positives* in a subsequent 3D detection network centered on regions of interest (ROIs). Although appropriate in the context of lung nodule detection, this is not the general case in medical imaging applications where false negative reduction is also, sometimes more so, of interest.

To this end, we develop a general deep learning framework that embeds uncertainty estimates across cascaded inference tasks in order to improve the performance of the downstream task of interest. Specifically, two different medical imaging contexts are investigated in which voxel-based uncertainty measures based on MC dropout (e.g. sample variance) are propagated to downstream tasks, where they are shown to improve network performance for the detection and segmentation of focal pathologies (e.g. lesions, tumours) in brain images by reducing both false positives *and* false negative predictions.

In the first context, a 3D fully-convolutional segmentation network is trained on a large multi-site, multi-scanner, proprietary dataset of MS patient MRI.

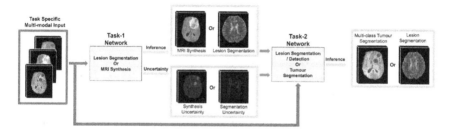

Fig. 1. Overview of the proposed general framework for propagating inference results and their associated uncertainties along sequential tasks in medical image analysis (Ex. MS T2 lesion segmentation, and MR synthesis - brain tumour segmentation). (Color figure online)

Segmentation uncertainty estimates are based on MC dropout sample variance. A second segmentation network is trained with this uncertainty as an additional input. Experimental results indicate that uncertainty propagation improves the T2 lesion true positive rate (TPR) from 0.78 to 0.84, in comparison to baseline (one stage network), at the clinically relevant false discovery rate (FDR) of 0.2. In the second context, a two-stage MR sequence synthesis and tumour segmentation pipeline is developed, which is trained and tested on the publicly available MICCAI 2018 BraTS dataset [13]. Experimental results indicate that propagating the synthesized image along with its associated uncertainty map to the downstream tumour segmentation network improves the Dice performance by anywhere from 2–10%, in comparison to only propagating synthesized image. Together, these contexts demonstrate that network uncertainty captures information supplementary to typical deterministic outputs, and can be successfully leveraged to improve the performance of downstream networks.

2 Methodology: Propagating Uncertainty Across Inference Tasks

An overview of the proposed method for propagating uncertainties across inference tasks is given in Fig. 1. The framework includes two different task specific networks, one for each of the sequential inference tasks, where each network takes images, here multi-modal MRI volumes, as inputs (blue arrows in Fig. 1). Task-1 produces the results of inference and their associated uncertainty values. In addition to MRI inputs, these outputs are provided to the Task-2 network as inputs (dark purple arrows in Fig. 1). We hypothesize that including the Task-1 network uncertainty output as an additional input to the Task-2 network will improve its performance.

The framework is general in that a number of methods can be used to estimate the uncertainties. In this work, the uncertainties produced by the Task-1 network are estimated using MC dropout sampling [7], where a network is trained using dropout and, during testing, the input is passed through the network with dropout N times to obtain N Monte-Carlo (MC) samples. The mean of these samples is taken as the network's output prediction, and the variance of the samples is used to estimate its uncertainty. Note that both the Task-1 network and the Task-2 network are trained separately. An end-to-end training of networks is not considered here as model uncertainties (resulting from MC-Dropout) on training cases would not properly reflect the model uncertainties on unseen test cases.

This work investigates two different pipelines, each of which cascades two different inference tasks. For the first pipeline, the Task-1 network consists of a Bayesian U-Net (BU-Net) [5], a segmentation network that takes multi-modal brain MRI of MS patients and produces a T2 lesion segmentation and a voxel-level uncertainty map. For the second pipeline, the Task-1 network is a synthesis network, which takes multi-modal MR sequences of patients with tumours (e.g. T1, T1ce, T2) as input and generates an additional unavailable MR sequence (e.g. FLAIR) along with the uncertainties for the regressed volume. For this task, the multi-task Regression-Segmentation Network (RS-Net) proposed in [2] is used.

The Task-2 network for both MS and brain tumour pipelines is a segmentation network which either results in MS T2 lesion segmentation or multi-class brain tumour segmentation, respectively. A modified 3D U-Net [12] is used for this task. Like the original 3D U-Net [12], the network consists of encoder and decoder paths that contain convolution, pooling, and up-sampling/deconvolution operations. High-resolution features from the encoder path are combined with the up-sampled output of decoder in an attempt to preserve high-resolution features. Each convolution is followed by non-linear activation (Leaky ReLU/ReLU). Instead of using the batch-normalization layer used in the original U-Net, we use group [14]/instance normalization [15]. This typically improves performance for small batch sizes. For MS T2 lesion segmentation, the network is trained using a combined, equally weighted Sorensen-Dice loss and binary cross-entropy loss, and produces binary lesion segmentation output. For tumour segmentation, the network is trained using categorical cross-entropy loss and produces multi-class tumour segmentation output.

3   Experiments and Results

For both MS T2 lesion segmentation and brain tumour segmentation pipelines, we investigate the network's performance in 3 settings: (1) Task-2 networks are trained on the same input MRI as Task-1, (2) In addition to MRI, the Task-2 network also takes the deterministic prediction of the Task-1 network as input, (3) MRI, deterministic predictions, and the uncertainty of the Task-1 network output are provided as input to the Task-2 network.

3.1   MS T2 Lesion Segmentation/Detection Pipeline

In this pipeline, both tasks consist of T2 lesion segmentation networks. For the first task, we train BU-Net [5] (Task-1 network) to segment T2 lesions given

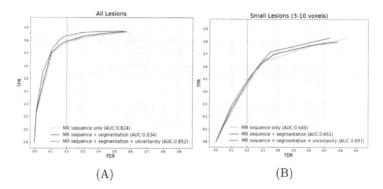

(A)   (B)

Fig. 2. Receiver-operating characteristic (ROC) curves comparing overall MS T2 lesion detection performance, illustrating TPR (true positive rate) vs. FDR (false detection rate) across (A) all lesions, and (B) small lesions (3–10 voxels) with several input configurations. At the operating point of FDR $= 0.2$, TPR values are (A) 0.44, 0.47, and 0.49 and (B) 0.78, 0.80, and 0.84 for MR sequence, MR sequence + segmentation, and MR sequence + segmentation + uncertainty experiments, respectively.

multiple MRI (T1, T2, FLAIR, and proton density (PD)), and provide a corresponding segmentation uncertainty. 10 Monte Carlo samples are used to compute the segmentation uncertainty. The second task consists of a modified 3D U-Net (Task-2 network) that again performs binary voxel-level T2 lesion segmentation. These voxel-level segmentations are subsequently grouped into discrete lesion-level instances.

A proprietary dataset, used for training and testing, consists of three multi-site, multi-scanner clinical relapsing-remitting MS (RRMS) trials, with a total of 2832 patients at different disease stages, resulting in over 5800 multi-modal MRI (T1, T2, FLAIR, and PD). The majority of these patients were scanned annually or bi-annually over a 24-month period. MRI sequences were acquired at 1 mm × 1 mm × 3 mm resolution. Expert T2 lesion labels provided with the dataset were the result of expert human annotators manually correcting an automated segmentation method. 40% of the available data was used for training/validating the Task-1 network, with a 90/10 training/validation split. 50% of the available data was used for training/validating the Task-2 network, again with a 90/10 training/validation split. Finally, 10% of the available data is used for testing the Task-2 network. The dataset is divided this way in order to provide the Task-2 network with consistent and meaningful uncertainties.

Since the downstream outcome of interest is the accurate detection of T2 lesions, we evaluate the performance of Task-1 and Task-2 networks based on lesion-level TPR and FDR. To obtain lesion-level detections from the voxel-based segmentations provided by the Task-2 network, a connected component analysis is performed to group lesion voxels together in an 18-connected neighbourhood [5]. The TPR and FDR are then calculated at the lesion level and are used to plot receiver operating characteristic (ROC) curves. Given that MS lesions

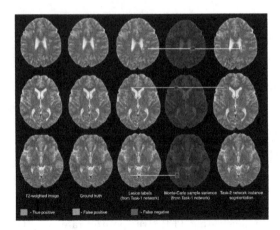

Fig. 3. Examples demonstrating the corrective effect of uncertainty propagation on MS lesion detection performance for three patients. Images are of, from left to right, T2 weighted MRI input, ground truth T2 lesion labels (in magenta), T2 lesion labels produced by the Task-1 network, the MC sample variance uncertainty estimates at the Task-1 network output, and the T2 lesion labels produced by the Task-2 network.

vary greatly in size, the system performance is evaluated on lesions grouped into three size bins: small (3–10 vox), medium (11–50 vox), and large (51+ vox). The system performs almost perfectly in detecting medium and large lesions in all 3 settings. Given that the detection of small lesions is particularly challenging, and that 40% of the lesions in the dataset are small, lesion detection ROC results are reported for both the overall performance on all lesions and then on only the small lesions in Fig. 2. At an FDR of 0.2 (the clinical operating point of interest), the TPR performance increases by 4% for small lesions and 5% for all lesions with the inclusion of the Task-1 uncertainty map as an additional input to the Task-2 network. Qualitative results for three cases are provided in Fig. 3 illustrate how the propagation of the uncertainty information enables the correction of both false positives (bottom case) and false negatives (top two cases).

3.2 Brain Tumour Segmentation Pipeline

Segmentation of brain tumours requires the presence of multiple MRI sequences (T1, T2, T1ce, and FLAIR) that provide complementary information. In clinical scenarios, one or more of these critical MR sequences might be missing (e.g. FLAIR), due to a variety of reasons, including cost or time constraints, noise in acquisition, etc. One way to address this is to synthesize the missing sequence before tumour segmentation [2,11]. We train RS-Net (Task-1 network) [2] to synthesize T1ce and FLAIR MRI, and generate its corresponding synthesis (regression) uncertainty. We synthesize these sequences as previous work [2,11] has shown that their absence will decrease segmentation performance more than the absence of either T1 or T2. T1ce is the hardest sequence to synthesize because

Table 1. Comparison of multi-class brain tumour segmentation based on modified 3D U-Net on the BraTS 2018 Validation dataset. The inclusion of the associated uncertainties from Task-1, in addition to the RS-Net synthesis output, as input to the 3D U-Net network is shown to lead to improvements on the Dice values. Quantitative segmentation results are based on percentage Dice coefficients for: enhancing tumor (DE), whole tumor (DT), and tumor core (DC). (*) indicates statistically significant (p ≤ 0.05) differences between second and third row.

	T1ce synthesis			FLR synthesis		
	DT	DC	DE	DT	DC	DE
real(3) sequences	87.17	50.25	26.89	83.27	73.91	71.07
real(3)+synthesized sequences	86.72	52.80	27.35	84.56	76.72	72.89
real(3)+synthesized+uncertainty	**88.20**	**57.29***	**32.86***	**85.84***	**79.25***	**74.51***

it shows enhancement within the tumour resulting from a contrast agent, which is not present in the other MRI sequences used in its synthesis. RS-Net uses T1, T2, and FLAIR to synthesize T1ce, and T1, T1ce, and T2 to synthesize FLAIR. Uncertainties associated with synthesized MRI are estimated using 20 MC samples. We then train a modified 3D U-Net (Task-2 network) for multi-class brain tumour segmentation, comparing three experiment settings detailed in Sect. 3.

This pipeline is evaluated using the 2018 MICCAI BraTS [13] dataset. The BraTS training dataset is comprised of 210 HGG and 75 LGG patients with different MRI sequences: T1, T1ce, T2, and FLAIR MRI for each patient. Ground truth tumour labels were provided by expert human annotators, and consist of 3 classes: edema, necrotic/non-enhancing core, and enhancing tumor core. 228 patients were randomly selected for training the network and another remaining 57 for network validation. A separate BraTS 2018 validation dataset was used to test the segmentation performance. This dataset contains 66 patient multi-channel MRI (with no labels provided). The BraTS challenge provides pre-processed volumes that were skull-stripped, co-aligned, and resampled to 1 mm × 1 mm × 1 mm voxel resolution. The intensities were additionally normalized using mean subtraction, divided by the standard deviation, and rescaled from 0 to 1, using the brain-masked region of a given MR image. The images were then cropped to $184 \times 200 \times 152$. To make sure that regression uncertainties are associated with data that was not seen during training, the RS-Net was trained in two folds, with each fold comprised of 114 volumes. The segmentation U-Net was trained using all 228 volumes in a single fold.

The performance of the brain tumour segmentation is evaluated by calculating Dice scores for three different tumour sub-types: enhancing tumour, whole tumour, and tumour core. This is consistent with the evaluation metrics used in the BraTS challenge [13]. Quantitative results (Table 1) indicate that when the associated regression uncertainty is propagated as an input to the segmentation (3D U-Net) network in addition to the synthesized MRI, the network performance increases by either 2–10% (T1ce synthesis) or 2–5% (FLAIR synthesis), over propagating only the synthesized MRI. As seen in other works [2,11] and

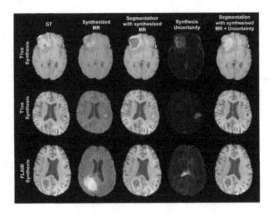

Fig. 4. Examples demonstrating the 3D U-Net performance on the multi-class brain tumour segmentation task based on synthesized MRI sequences. From Left to Right: GT segmentation, synthesized MR sequence, segmentation using real MRI (3 sequences) + synthesized MRI, synthesis uncertainty, segmentation using real MRI (3 sequences) + synthesized MRI + synthesis uncertainty. First two rows: T1ce synthesis. Last row: FLAIR synthesis. Labels: edema (green), non-enhancing or necrotic tumour core (red), enhancing tumour (yellow). (Color figure online)

mentioned above, the overall network performance is lower for T1ce as compared to FLAIR as it is more challenging to synthesize.

Figure 4 shows visual examples of the results on the downstream brain tumour segmentation when MRI sequences are synthesized. In the first row, it is clear that the framework that does not include synthesis uncertainty results in confusion between enhancing tumour and core tumour, as the enhancement is not well captured in the synthesized T1ce. However, the synthesis uncertainty is higher in this region. Consequently, propagating the uncertainty information informs the Task-2 (segmentation) network about mistakes made by Task-1 (synthesis) network, thereby enabling the correction of these errors. Similarly, in the second row, we can see that uncertainty provides supplementary information to the synthesized T1ce and allows the network to correctly identify enhancing and non-enhancing core. In the third row, the FLAIR sequence is synthesized. Here, the network incorrectly segments background near and within the ventricle as edema when uncertainty is not propagated. This is because the ventricle is incorrectly highlighted in this area in the synthesized FLAIR. As the uncertainty for this synthesized region is high, cascading the uncertainties permits the network to learn to correct its error.

4   Conclusions

This work proposes a general deep learning framework for the propagation of uncertainty across a sequence of inference tasks within a medical image analysis pipeline, and demonstrated that cascading uncertainties (e.g. based on MC dropout) in this manner can lead to improvements in performance for the downstream task. The framework was applied to two different contexts. First, it was demonstrated that by propagating voxel-based lesion segmentation uncertainties to a second segmentation network, lesion-level detection performance can be improved (in terms of a reduction of both FPs and FNs) based on experiments on a large-scale, multi-site, clinical dataset of patients with MS. Next, it was also demonstrated that by propagating regression uncertainty from an MRI synthesis task, performance of a downstream multi-class tumour segmentation task can be improved based on experiments on the publicly available BraTS dataset. Future work will explore how to properly develop a complete end-to-end system that includes uncertainty propagation across the inference modules.

Acknowledgements. This work was supported by a Canadian Natural Science and Engineering Research Council (NSERC) Collaborative Research and Development Grant (CRDPJ 505357 - 16), Synaptive Medical, the Canadian NSERC Discovery and CREATE grants, and an award from the International Progressive MS Alliance (PA-1603-08175).

References

1. Chartsias, A., Joyce, T., Giuffrida, M.V., Tsaftaris, S.A.: Multimodal MR synthesis via modality-invariant latent representation. IEEE Trans. Med. Imaging **37**(3), 803–814 (2017)
2. Mehta, R., Arbel, T.: RS-Net: regression-segmentation 3D CNN for synthesis of full resolution missing brain MRI in the presence of tumours. In: Gooya, A., Goksel, O., Oguz, I., Burgos, N. (eds.) SASHIMI 2018. LNCS, pp. 119–129. Springer, Cham (2018). https://doi.org/10.1007/978-3-030-00536-8_13
3. Dalca, A.V., Balakrishnan, G., Guttag, J., Sabuncu, M.R.: Unsupervised learning for fast probabilistic diffeomorphic registration. In: Frangi, A.F., Schnabel, J.A., Davatzikos, C., Alberola-López, C., Fichtinger, G. (eds.) MICCAI 2018. LNCS, vol. 11070, pp. 729–738. Springer, Cham (2018). https://doi.org/10.1007/978-3-030-00928-1_82
4. Isensee, F., Kickingereder, P., Wick, W., Bendszus, M., Maier-Hein, K.H.: No new-net. In: Crimi, A., Bakas, S., Kuijf, H., Keyvan, F., Reyes, M., van Walsum, T. (eds.) BrainLes 2018. LNCS, vol. 11384, pp. 234–244. Springer, Cham (2019). https://doi.org/10.1007/978-3-030-11726-9_21
5. Nair, T., Precup, D., Arnold, D.L., Arbel, T.: Exploring uncertainty measures in deep networks for multiple sclerosis lesion detection and segmentation. In: Frangi, A.F., Schnabel, J.A., Davatzikos, C., Alberola-López, C., Fichtinger, G. (eds.) MICCAI 2018. LNCS, vol. 11070, pp. 655–663. Springer, Cham (2018). https://doi.org/10.1007/978-3-030-00928-1_74
6. Tousignant, A., Lemaître, P., Precup, D., Arnold, D.L., Arbel, T.: Prediction of disease progression in multiple sclerosis patients using deep learning analysis of MRI data. In: International Conference on Medical Imaging with Deep Learning, pp. 483–492, May 2019
7. Gal, Y., Ghahramani, Z.: Dropout as a Bayesian approximation: representing model uncertainty in deep learning. In: International Conference on Machine Learning, pp. 1050–1059, June 2016

8. Ozdemir, O., Woodward, B., Berlin, A.A.: Propagating uncertainty in multi-stage Bayesian convolutional neural networks with application to pulmonary nodule detection. arXiv preprint arXiv:1712.00497 (2017)
9. Roy, A.G., Conjeti, S., Navab, N., Wachinger, C., Alzheimer's Disease Neuroimaging Initiative: Bayesian QuickNAT: model uncertainty in deep whole-brain segmentation for structure-wise quality control. NeuroImage **195**, 11–22 (2019)
10. Leibig, C., Allken, V., Ayhan, M.S., Berens, P., Wahl, S.: Leveraging uncertainty information from deep neural networks for disease detection. Sci. Rep. **7**(1), 17816 (2017)
11. van Tulder, G., de Bruijne, M.: Why does synthesized data improve multi-sequence classification? In: Navab, N., Hornegger, J., Wells, W.M., Frangi, A.F. (eds.) MICCAI 2015. LNCS, vol. 9349, pp. 531–538. Springer, Cham (2015). https://doi.org/10.1007/978-3-319-24553-9_65
12. Çiçek, Ö., Abdulkadir, A., Lienkamp, S.S., Brox, T., Ronneberger, O.: 3D U-Net: learning dense volumetric segmentation from sparse annotation. In: Ourselin, S., Joskowicz, L., Sabuncu, M.R., Unal, G., Wells, W. (eds.) MICCAI 2016. LNCS, vol. 9901, pp. 424–432. Springer, Cham (2016). https://doi.org/10.1007/978-3-319-46723-8_49
13. Bakas, S., et al.: Identifying the best machine learning algorithms for brain tumor segmentation, progression assessment, and overall survival prediction in the BRATS challenge. arXiv preprint arXiv:1811.02629 (2018)
14. Wu, Y., He, K.: Group normalization. In: Ferrari, V., Hebert, M., Sminchisescu, C., Weiss, Y. (eds.) ECCV 2018. LNCS, vol. 11217, pp. 3–19. Springer, Cham (2018). https://doi.org/10.1007/978-3-030-01261-8_1
15. Ulyanov, D., Vedaldi, A., Lempitsky, V.: Instance normalization: the missing ingredient for fast stylization. arXiv preprint arXiv:1607.08022 (2016)

Reg R-CNN: Lesion Detection and Grading Under Noisy Labels

Gregor N. Ramien$^{(\boxtimes)}$, Paul F. Jaeger, Simon A. A. Kohl,
and Klaus H. Maier-Hein

Division of Medical Image Computing, German Cancer Research Center (DKFZ),
Heidelberg, Germany
g.ramien@dkfz.de

Abstract. For the task of concurrently detecting and categorizing objects, the medical imaging community commonly adopts methods developed on natural images. Current state-of-the-art object detectors are comprised of two stages: the first stage generates region proposals, the second stage subsequently categorizes them. Unlike in natural images, however, for anatomical structures of interest such as tumors, the appearance in the image (e.g., scale or intensity) links to a malignancy grade that lies on a continuous *ordinal scale*. While classification models discard this ordinal relation between grades by discretizing the continuous scale to an unordered bag of categories, regression models are trained with distance metrics, which preserve the relation. This advantage becomes all the more important in the setting of label confusions on ambiguous data sets, which is the usual case with medical images. To this end, we propose Reg R-CNN, which replaces the second-stage classification model of a current object detector with a regression model. We show the superiority of our approach on a public data set with 1026 patients and a series of toy experiments. Code will be available at github.com/MIC-DKFZ/RegRCNN.

Keywords: Lesion detection · Malignancy grading · Noisy labels

1 Introduction

The task of concurrently detecting and categorizing objects has been extensively studied in classic computer vision [5,12]. In medical image computing, numerous approaches have been proposed to predict lesion locations and gradings, most of them in a supervised manner utilizing manual annotations. However, when adopting state-of-the-art object detectors for end-to-end lesion grading, one has to account for an inherent difference in the data: The grading of lesions denotes a subjective discretization of naturally continuous and ordered features (such as

---

S.A.A. Kohl—Now with the Karlsruhe Institute of Technology and DeepMind (London).

© Springer Nature Switzerland AG 2019
H. Greenspan et al. (Eds.): CLIP 2019/UNSURE 2019, LNCS 11840, pp. 33–41, 2019.
https://doi.org/10.1007/978-3-030-32689-0_4

scale or intensity) to semantic categories with clinical meaning (e.g., BI-RADS score, Gleason score [14], PI-RADS score, TNM staging). This is in contrast to typical tasks on natural images, where categories can be described as an unordered set (no natural ordinal relation exists between dogs and cars). Hence, current object detectors phrase the categorization as a classification task and are trained using the cross-entropy loss, not considering the continuous ordinal relation between classes (see Sect. 2.1).

In this paper, we account for the ordinal information in lesion appearance and derived categories, aiming to improve model performance. To this end, we propose Reg R-CNN, which replaces the classification model of Mask R-CNN [5], a state-of-the-art object detector, with a regression model. Regression models utilize distance metrics, i.e., models are trained directly on the underlying continuous scale, which has the following major benefit in the setting of lesion grading on medical images:

Medical data sets often exhibit high ambiguity that is reflected in the variability of the human annotations. Under the assumption that class confusions follow a distribution around the underlying ground truth, distance metrics used in regression such as the L1-distance are more tolerant to mild deviation from the target value as opposed to the categorical cross entropy which penalizes all off-target predictions in equal measure [4].

We empirically show the superiority of Reg R-CNN on a public data set with 1026 patients and a series of toy experiments with code made publicly available.

2   Methods

2.1   Regression vs. Classification Training

In order to see why we expect the training of regression models to be more robust to label noise than classification models for the case when target classes lie on a continuous scale, let us first revisit the objective commonly minimized by classifiers. This objective is the cross entropy (CE), defined as

$$H\left(\mathbf{p}, \mathbf{q}; \mathbf{X}\right) = -\sum_{j} p_j(\mathbf{X}) \log q_j(\mathbf{X}) \tag{1}$$

between a target distribution $\mathbf{p}(\mathbf{X})$ over discrete labels $j \in C$ and the predicted distribution $\mathbf{q}(\mathbf{X})$ given data $\mathbf{X}$. For mutually exclusive classes, the target distribution is given by a delta distribution $\mathbf{p}(\mathbf{X}) = \{\delta_{ij}\}_{j \in C}$.

To produce a prediction $\mathbf{q}(\mathbf{X})$, the network's logits $\mathbf{z}(\mathbf{X})$ are squashed by means of a softmax function:

$$\mathbf{q}(\mathbf{X}) = \frac{e^{\mathbf{z}(\mathbf{X})}}{\sum_{k \in C} e^{z_k(\mathbf{X})}}, \tag{2}$$

which, plugged into Eq. 1 and given the target class i, leads to the loss term

$$H = \mathcal{L}_{CE}(\mathbf{p} = \delta_{ij}, \mathbf{q}; \mathbf{X}) = -z_i + log \sum_k e^{z_k}. \tag{3}$$

From Eq. 3 it is apparent that the standard CE loss treats labels as an unordered bag of targets, where all off-target classes ($j \neq i$) are penalized in equal measure, regardless of their proximity to the target class i. Distance metrics on the other hand, as their name suggests, take into account the distance of a prediction to the target. This lets the loss scale in the deviation of prediction to target. Allowing to be more accepting of mild discrepancies, it better accommodates for noise from potentially conflicting labels in settings where the target labels lie on a continuum.

In the range of experiments below, we compare classification against regression setups, for which we employed the smooth L1 loss [6] given by

$$\mathcal{L}_{reg}(p, t) = \begin{cases} 1/2(t - p)^2, & |t - p| < 1 \\ |t - p| - 1/2, & \text{otherwise} \end{cases} \tag{4}$$

for predicted value p and target value t. Other works have investigated adaptions to the CE loss to account for noisy labels in classification tasks, e.g. [15,17]. Our approach is complementary to those works as it exploits label continua on medical images.

2.2 Reg R-CNN and Baseline

The proposed Reg R-CNN architecture is based on Mask R-CNN [5], a state-of-the-art two-stage detector. In Mask R-CNN, first, objects are discriminated from background irrespective of class, accompanied by bounding-box regression to generate region proposals of variable sizes. Second, proposals are resampled to a fixed-sized grid and fed through three head networks: A classifier for categorization, a second bounding-box regressor for refinement of coordinates, and a fully convolutional head producing output segmentations (the latter are not further used in this study except for the additional pixel-wise loss during training). Reg R-CNN (see Fig. 1) simply replaces the classification head by a regression head, which is trained with the smooth L1 loss instead of the cross-entropy loss (see Sect. 2.1).

For the final filtering of output predictions, non-maximum suppression (NMS) is performed based on detection-confidence scores. In Mask R-CNN, these are provided by the classification head. Since the regression head does not produce confidences, we use the objectness scores from the first stage instead.

In this study, we compare Reg R-CNN against Mask R-CNN as the classification counterpart of our approach. Only minor changes are made with respect to the original publication [5]: The number of feature maps in the region proposal network is lowered to 64 to account for GPU memory constraints. The poolsize of 3D RoIAlign (a 3D re-implementation of the resampling method used to create fixed-sized proposals) is set to (7, 7, 3) for the classification head and (14, 14, 5) for the mask head. The matching Intersection over Union (IoU) for positive proposals is lowered to 0.3. Objectness scores are used for the final NMS to reflect the desired disentanglement of detection and categorization tasks.

Note that all changes apply to Reg R-CNN as well, such that the only difference between the models is the exchange of the classification head with a regression head.

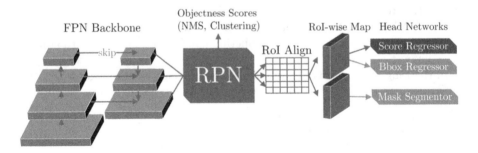

Fig. 1. Reg R-CNN for joint detection and grading of objects. The architecture is closely related to Mask R-CNN [5], where grading is done with a classification head instead of the displayed "Score Regressor" head network. FPN denotes the feature pyramid network [11], RPN denotes the region proposal network and RoIAlign is the operation which resamples object proposals to a fixed-sized grid before categorization.

2.3   Evaluation

Comparing the performance of regression to classification models requires taking into account additional considerations since both are trained along an upstream detection task.

In order to compare continuous regression and discrete classification outputs, we bin the continuous regression output after training, such that bin centers match the discrete classification targets.

What's more, the joint task of object detection and categorization is commonly evaluated using average precision (AP) [2]. However, AP requires per-category confidence scores, which are, as mentioned before, not provided by regression outputs. Instead, we borrow a metric commonly used in viewpoint estimation, the Average Viewpoint Precision (AVP) [16]. Based on AVP, we phrase the lesion scoring as an additional task on top of foreground vs. background object detection: In order for a box prediction to be considered a true positive, it needs to match the ground-truth box with an IoU > 0.1[1], and additionally the malignancy prediction score is required to lie in the correct category bin. This way, AVP simultaneously measures both the detection and malignancy-scoring performance of the models. We additionally disentangle the task performances and separately report the AP of foreground vs. background detection (this poses an upper bound on AVP) and the bin accuracy. The latter is determined by selecting only true positive predictions according to the detection metric and counting malignancy-score matches with the target bin.

---

[1] This relatively low matching threshold respects the clinical need for coarse localization and exploits the non-overlapping nature of objects in 3D images.

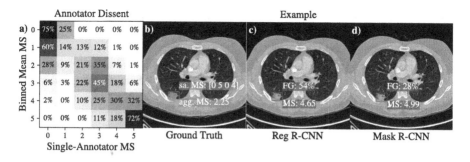

Fig. 2. (a) A confusion-matrix-style display of annotator dissent in the LIDC data set. Rows represent the binned mean ratings of lesions (in place of the true class in a standard confusion matrix), columns the ratings of the corresponding single annotators. "MS" means malignancy score. Matrix is row-wisely normalized, hence cell values indicate distribution of lesion ratings within a bin. **(b)–(d)** Example slice from the LIDC data set showing GT, Reg R-CNN, and Mask R-CNN prediction separately. GT note "sa. MS" shows the single-annotator grades (grade 0 means no finding), "agg. MS" their mean. In the predictions, "FG" means foreground confidence (objectness score), "MS" denotes the predicted malignancy score. Mask R-CNN MS can be non-integer due to Weighted Box Clustering [7]. Color symbolizes bin.

3   Experiments

3.1   Utilized Data Sets

Lung CT Data Set. The utilized LIDC-IDRI data set consists of 1026 patients with annotations of four medical experts each [1]. Having disposable multiple gradings from distinct annotators is a rare exception on medical images and allows to investigate the exhibited label noise [9].

Full agreement, which we define as all raters assigning the same malignancy label to all lesions (RoIs) in a patient, is observed on a mere 163 patients (this includes patients void of findings by all raters). This corresponds to a rater disagreement with respect to the malignancy scoring on 84% of the patients. On a lesion level (RoI-wise), the data set comprises 2631 lesions when considering all lesions with a positive label by at least one rater. This number drops to 1834, 1333, or 821, when requiring 2, 3, or 4 positive labels respectively. This shows that this data set's labelling is both ambiguous with respect to whether or not a lesion is present as well as the prospective lesion's grading. The first ambiguity type has bearings on the detection head's performance, while the second type influences the network's classification or, respectively, regression head.

In order to evaluate the grading performance, the following malignancy statistics include only patients with at least one finding. Among those, we count 99 lesions (3.8% of all lesions) with full rater agreement, leaving disagreement on 2532 (or 96.2%). The standard deviation of the 4 graders averaged over all lesions amounts to 1.05 malignancy-score values (ms). In Fig. 2(a), we show how the single graders' malignancy ratings differ given the binned mean rating. The figure reveals significant label confusion across adjacent labels and even beyond. Figures 2(b)–(d) display example Reg and Mask R-CNN predictions next to the corresponding ground truth.

In order to investigate the models' performance under label noise, we randomly sample a malignancy score (MS) for a given lesion from the 4 given gradings at each training iteration. At test time, we however employ the lesions' mean malignancy score as the ground truth label, which allows to evaluate against a ground truth of reduced noise.

Toy Data Set. To analyze the performance of Reg R-CNN vs. Mask R-CNN on an artificial data set with label noise on a continuous scale, we designed a set of 3D toy images. The associated task is the joint detection and categorization of cylinders, where five categories are distinguished as cylinders of five different radii. In order to simulate label confusion, Gaussian noise is added to the isotropic target radii during training, sampled with standard deviation $\sigma = r/6$ around object radius r, as depicted in Figs. 3(c) and (d). This causes targets (especially of large-radius objects) to be shifted into wrong, yet mostly adjacent target bins. Figure 3(a) portrays that these ambiguities are imprinted on the images as a belt of reduced intensity with width 2σ around the actual radius. At test time, model predictions are evaluated against the exact target radii without noise. The data set consists of 1.5k randomly generated samples for training and validation, as well as a hold-out test set of 1k images.

3.2 Training and Inference Setup

Both the LIDC and the toy data set consist of volumetric images. In this study, we evaluate models both in 3D as well as 2D (slice-wise processing). For the sake of comparability, all methods are implemented in a single framework and run with identical hyperparameters. Networks are trained on patch crops of sizes $160 \times 160 \times 96$ (LIDC) and $320 \times 320 \times 8$ (toy), oversampling of foreground regions is applied. Class imbalances in object-level classification losses are accounted for by stochastically mining the hardest negative object candidates according to softmax probability.

On LIDC, models are trained for 130 epochs, each composed of 200 batches with size 8 (20) in 3D (2D) using the Adam optimizer [8] with default settings at a learning rate of 10^{-4}. Training is performed as a five-fold cross validation (splits: train 60%/val 20%/test 20%). At test time, we ensemble the four best performing models according to validation metrics over four test-time views (three mirroring augmentations) in each fold. Aggregation of box predictions from ensemble members is done via clustering and weighted averaging of scores and coordinates. Predictions from 2D models are consolidated along the z-axis by means of an adaption of NMS and evaluated against the 3D ground truth.

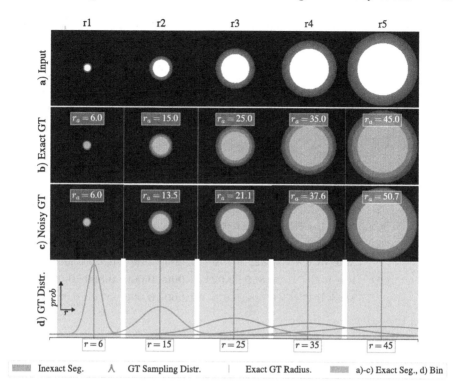

Fig. 3. (a) Cylinders (2D projections) of all five categories (r1-r5) in the toy experiment. (b) Exact GT. (c) Examples of a noisy GT for each category (r1-r5). r_a indicates the annotated radius (target regression value). (d) Gaussian sampling distributions used to generate the noisy GT. Green vertical lines depict the exact ground-truth values, while blue lines are the corresponding label-noise distributions. Green rectangles are the bins (borders enlarged for illustration) used for training of the classifier as well as for evaluation of both methods. Note that distributions reach into neighboring bins leading to label confusions. (Color figure online)

3.3 Results and Discussion

Results are shown in Table 1. In addition to the fold means of the metrics, we report the corresponding standard deviations. On LIDC, Reg R-CNN outperforms Mask R-CNN on both input dimensions and all three considered metrics. On the toy data set, Reg R-CNN shows superior performance in AVP_{10} and Bin Accuracy. AP_{10} reaches 100% in both models indicating that the detection task is solved entirely, i.e., the object grading task has been isolated successfully (hence, results for AVP_{10} converge towards the Bin Accuracy). All experiments demonstrate the superiority of distance losses in the supervision of models performing continuous and ordered grading under noisy labels. Interestingly, there is a marked increase in performance for both setups when running in 3D as opposed to 2D, suggesting that additional 3D context is generally beneficial for the task.

Table 1. Results for LIDC and the toy data set. AVP_{10} measures joint detection and categorization performance, while AP_{10} measures the disentangled detection performance and Bin Accuracy shows categorization performance (conditioned on detection, see Sect. 2.3)

	Dim	Network head	AVP_{10}	AP_{10}	Bin accuracy
LIDC	3D	Reg R-CNN	**0.259±0.035**	**0.628±0.038**	**0.477±0.035**
		Mask R-CNN	0.235±0.027	0.622±0.029	0.411±0.026
	2D	Reg R-CNN	**0.148±0.046**	**0.414±0.052**	**0.468±0.057**
		Mask R-CNN	0.127±0.034	0.406±0.040	0.447±0.018
Toy	3D	Reg R-CNN	**0.881±0.014**	0.998±0.004	**0.887±0.014**
		Mask R-CNN	0.822±0.070	**1.000±.000**	0.826±0.069
	2D	Reg R-CNN	**0.859±0.021**	**1.000±0.000**	**0.860±0.021**
		Mask R-CNN	0.748±0.022	**1.000±0.000**	0.748±0.021

4   Conclusion

Simultaneously detecting and grading objects is a common and clinically highly relevant task in medical image analysis. As opposed to natural images, where object categories are mostly well defined, the categorizations of interest for clinically relevant findings commonly leave room for interpretation. This ambiguity can bear on machine-learning models in the form of noisy labels, which may hamper the performance of classification models. Clinical label categories however often reside on a continuous and ordered scale, suggesting that label confusions are likely more frequent between adjacent categories.

For this case, we show that both the performance of lesion detection and malignancy grading can be improved upon over a state-of-the-art detection model when simply trading its classification for a regression head and altering the loss accordingly. We document the success of the ensuing model Reg R-CNN on a large lung CT data set and on a toy data set that induces artificial ambiguity. We attribute the edge in performance to the loss formulation of the regression task, which naturally accounts for the continuous relation between labels and is therefore less prone to suffer from conflicting gradients from noisy labels.

5   Outlook

As Eq. 4 shows, we employ a metric approach to ordinal data. In general, this is not hazard-free as model performance may suffer from the imposed metric if the scale actually is non-metric [10]. In other words, our approach implicitly assumes the grading scale has sufficiently metric-like properties. To address this limitation, we plan to study alternative non-metric approaches in future work [3,13].

References

1. Armato III, S., et al.: Data from LIDC-IDRI. the cancer imaging archive
2. Everingham, M., Van Gool, L., Williams, C.K.I., Winn, J., Zisserman, A.: The pascal visual object classes (voc) challenge. IJCV **88**(2), 303–338 (2010)
3. Feindt, M.: A neural bayesian estimator for conditional probability densities. arXiv preprint physics/0402093 (2004)
4. Ghosh, A., Kumar, H., Sastry, P.: Robust loss functions under label noise for deep neural networks. In: Thirty-First AAAI Conference on Artificial Intelligence (2017)
5. He, K., Gkioxari, G., Dollár, P., Girshick, R.: Mask R-CNN. In: ICCV, pp. 2980–2988. IEEE (2017)
6. Huber, P.J.: Robust estimation of a location parameter. Ann. Math. Stat. **35**(1), 73101 (1964)
7. Jaeger, P.F., et al.: Retina u-net: embarrassingly simple exploitation of segmentation supervision for medical object detection. CoRR, abs/1811.08661 (2018)
8. Kingma, D.P., Ba, J.: Adam: A method for stochastic optimization. arXiv preprint arXiv:1412.6980 (2014)
9. Kohl, S., et al.: A probabilistic u-net for segmentation of ambiguous images. In: NIPS, pp. 6965–6975 (2018)
10. Liddell, T.M., Kruschke, J.K.: Analyzing ordinal data with metric models: what could possibly go wrong? J. Exp. Soc. Psychol. **79**, 328–348 (2018)
11. Lin, T.-Y., Dollár, P., Girshick, R.B., He, K., Hariharan, B., Belongie, S.J.: Feature pyramid networks for object detection. In: CVPR, vol. 1, p. 4 (2017)
12. Lin, T.-Y., Goyal, P., Girshick, R., He, K., Dollár, P.: Focal loss for dense object detection. In: TPAMI (2018)
13. McCullagh, P.: Regression models for ordinal data. J. Roy. Stat. Soc.: Ser. B (Methodol.) **42**(2), 109–127 (1980)
14. Nagpal, K., et al.: Development and validation of a deep learning algorithm for improving gleason scoring of prostate cancer. arXiv preprint arXiv:1811.06497 (2018)
15. Tanno, R., Saeedi, A., Sankaranarayanan, S., Alexander, D.C., Silberman, N.: Learning From Noisy Labels By Regularized Estimation Of Annotator Confusion. arXiv e-prints, page arXiv:1902.03680, February 2019
16. Xiang, Y., Mottaghi, R., Savarese, S.: Beyond pascal: a benchmark for 3D object detection in the wild. In: WACV (2014)
17. Zhang, Z., Sabuncu, M.R.: Generalized cross entropy loss for training deep neural networks with noisy labels. CoRR, abs/1805.07836 (2018)

Fast Nonparametric Mutual-Information-based Registration and Uncertainty Estimation

Mikael Agn[1(✉)] and Koen Van Leemput[1,2]

[1] Department of Health Technology, Technical University of Denmark,
Lyngby, Denmark
miag@dtu.dk
[2] Martinos Center for Biomedical Imaging, MGH, Harvard Medical School,
Boston, USA

Abstract. In this paper we propose a probabilistic model for multi-modal non-linear registration that directly incorporates the mutual information (MI) metric into a demons-like optimization scheme. In contrast to uni-modal registration, where the demons algorithm uses repeated spatial filtering to obtain very fast solutions, MI-based registration currently relies on general-purpose optimization schemes that are much slower. The central idea of this work is to reformulate an often-used histogram interpolation technique in MI implementations as an explicit spatial interpolation step within a generative model. By exploiting the specific structure of this model, we obtain a dedicated and fast expectation-maximization optimizer with demons-like properties. This also leads to an easy-to-implement Gibbs sampler to infer registration uncertainty in high-dimensional deformation models, involving very little additional code and no external tuning. Preliminary experiments on multi-modal brain MRI images show that the proposed optimizer can be both faster and more accurate than the free-form deformation method implemented in Elastix. We also demonstrate the sampler's ability to produce direct uncertainty estimates of MI-based registrations – to the best of our knowledge the first method in the literature to do so.

1 Introduction

An accurate and efficient way of non-linearly aligning two images with similar contrast properties is to minimize the sum-of-squared-differences (SSD) between them. The properties of the SSD criterion can be exploited to yield a dedicated optimization algorithm, the so-called demons algorithm [1,2], which repeatedly computes deformation "votes" at each voxel location, and spatially filters these votes to yield a spatially consistent deformation field. This results in fast optimizations of highly flexible, nonparametric deformation fields, taking only a few minutes on a standard desktop computer. Furthermore, the SSD criterion can

© Springer Nature Switzerland AG 2019
H. Greenspan et al. (Eds.): CLIP 2019/UNSURE 2019, LNCS 11840, pp. 42–51, 2019.
https://doi.org/10.1007/978-3-030-32689-0_5

be cast within a probabilistic modeling framework, making it possible to quantify registration uncertainty by approximating the relevant posterior probability
distributions, using either variational [3–6] or sampling [7–10] methods.

In contrast to these methodological advances in deformable uni-modal registration, the *de facto* standard in the field of multi-modal registration using
mutual information (MI) remains the free-form deformation approach [11],
in which a parametric deformation model of B-spline basis functions is optimized with general-purpose optimization algorithms (e.g., [12,13]). This approach yields accurate registration results, but at a considerable computational
cost when deformations with many degrees of freedom are needed (small spacing
between the B-spline knots). Although attempts have been made to adapt faster,
demons-like optimization schemes to the MI criterion [14–16], these methods
have merely replaced the SSD-based demons "votes" with spatial MI gradients,
a heuristic that does not necessarily optimize any specific objective function.
Unlike the SSD criterion, MI does not currently have an associated probabilistic
model [17], and consequently no principled way to quantify registration uncertainty.

In order to bring the SSD-specific techniques for uncertainty estimation and
fast, nonparametric registration into the realm of MI-based registration, the contribution of this paper is threefold. First, we show that the partial volume interpolation technique for computing MI using fractional histogram counts [18,19]
can be re-cast as a generative probabilistic model with an explicit spatial interpolation model. Second, we derive a tailor-made optimization algorithm that
makes judicious use of latent variables in this model to obtain local "votes" of
voxel-wise deformations that are subsequently regularized, allowing for a similar efficient optimization of nonparametric deformation models as in the demons
algorithm. And third, using largely the same code base as the proposed optimizer,
we also derive a practical technique for Monte Carlo sampling from the registration posterior, allowing for direct visualization and quantification of uncertainty
in MI-based models. In contrast to existing methods for uncertainty estimation in uni-modal registration [3–10], this sampler does not involve variational
approximations that may significantly underestimate uncertainty [9]; does not
require tuning of various Metropolis-Hastings proposal distribution parameters;
and can readily handle full 3D nonparametric deformation models with orders-
of-magnitude more degrees of freedom than the sparse models used so far.

2 Generative Model

Let $\mathbf{u} = (u_1, \ldots, u_I)^\mathrm{T}$ denote an image with I voxels, where the intensities
$u_i \in \{1, \ldots, L\}$ can take L discrete values. We model $\mathbf{u}$ as being generated from
another image $\mathbf{v} = (v_1, \ldots, v_J)^\mathrm{T}$ with J voxels that we will refer to as "nodes",
with intensities $v_j \in \{1, \ldots, K\}$ taken from K discrete levels, which we will call
"classes". This is achieved by associating with each voxel i a spatial deformation
d_i that maps that voxel to a spatial location $x_i + d_i$ in $\mathbf{v}$, where x_i denotes the
voxel's initial position in $\mathbf{v}$. We also associate with each class k a class-specific

intensity distribution parameterized by $\boldsymbol{\theta}_k = (\theta_{k,1}, \ldots, \theta_{k,L})^{\mathrm{T}}$, where $\theta_{k,l}$ denotes the probability that the kth class generates an intensity with value l. In the remainder, we assume periodic boundary conditions, and we only present the case in 1D, although the extension to higher dimensions is straightforward.

Using the notation $\mathbf{d} = (d_1, \ldots, d_I)^{\mathrm{T}}$ and $\boldsymbol{\theta} = \{\boldsymbol{\theta}_k\}_{k=1}^{K}$ for the deformation field and the collection of all intensity distribution parameters, respectively, the generative process of $\mathbf{u}$ proceeds as follows: Let $\mathbf{n} = (n_1, \ldots, n_I)^{\mathrm{T}}$, $n_i \in \{1, \ldots, J\}$ denote latent node assignments, whereby each voxel i is associated with one node by centering a bth order B-spline $\beta^b(\cdot)$ around its deformed position $x_i + d_i$, and using the B-spline value at each node location as the probability of that node being selected:

$$p(\mathbf{n}|\mathbf{d}) = \prod_{i=1}^{I} p(n_i|\mathbf{d}), \quad p(n_i = j|\mathbf{d}) = \beta^b(y_j - (x_i + d_i)),$$

where y_j denotes the spatial location of the jth node. Subsequently, an intensity is drawn in each voxel from the distribution associated with the class of the selected node:

$$p(\mathbf{u}|\mathbf{n}, \boldsymbol{\theta}) = \prod_{i=1}^{I} p(u_i|n_i, \boldsymbol{\theta}), \quad p(u_i|n_i = j, \boldsymbol{\theta}) = \theta_{v_j, u_i}.$$

This induces a marginal distribution

$$p(\mathbf{u}|\mathbf{d}, \boldsymbol{\theta}) = \sum_{\mathbf{n}} p(\mathbf{u}|\mathbf{n}, \boldsymbol{\theta}) p(\mathbf{n}|\mathbf{d}) = \prod_{i=1}^{I} \left(\sum_{k=1}^{K} \pi_k(x_i + d_i) \theta_{k, u_i} \right)$$

where $\pi_k(z) = \sum_{j=1}^{J} [v_j = k] \beta^b(z - y_j)$ is a spatial map of the probability of class k, obtained as a B-spline expansion of the class assignments in the nodes of $\mathbf{v}$. Thus, the model effectively generates $\mathbf{u}$ by drawing, in each voxel i, a class from these probabilistic maps at location $x_i + d_i$, and subsequently generating an intensity from the selected class-specific intensity distribution.

The model is completed by specifying a prior encouraging spatial smoothness in the deformation field $p(\mathbf{d}) \propto \exp\left(-\frac{\gamma}{2}\|\boldsymbol{\Gamma}\mathbf{d}\|^2\right)$, where $\boldsymbol{\Gamma}$ is a $I \times I$ circulant matrix implementing a high-pass filter, and a prior $p(\boldsymbol{\theta}) = \prod_{k=1}^{K} \mathrm{Dir}(\boldsymbol{\theta}_k|\boldsymbol{\alpha}_0)$, where $\mathrm{Dir}(\cdot|\boldsymbol{\alpha}_0)$ denotes the Dirichlet distribution with parameters $\boldsymbol{\alpha}_0$. (A flat prior $p(\boldsymbol{\theta}) \propto 1$ is obtained by choosing $\boldsymbol{\alpha}_0 = \mathbf{1}$.)

3 Optimization

Registration of $\mathbf{u}$ with $\mathbf{v}$ can be obtained by fitting the model to the data: $(\hat{\mathbf{d}}, \hat{\boldsymbol{\theta}}) = \arg\max_{(\mathbf{d}, \boldsymbol{\theta})} p(\mathbf{d}, \boldsymbol{\theta}|\mathbf{u})$ where $p(\mathbf{d}, \boldsymbol{\theta}|\mathbf{u}) \propto p(\mathbf{u}|\mathbf{d}, \boldsymbol{\theta}) p(\mathbf{d}) p(\boldsymbol{\theta})$. For this purpose, we propose an expectation-maximization (EM) algorithm that exploits the latent node assignments $\mathbf{n}$ in the model to achieve an efficient optimization strategy. In particular, we iteratively increase $\log p(\mathbf{d}, \boldsymbol{\theta}|\mathbf{u})$ from the current parameter estimates $(\tilde{\mathbf{d}}, \tilde{\boldsymbol{\theta}})$ by considering a lower bound $Q(\mathbf{d}, \boldsymbol{\theta}|\tilde{\mathbf{d}}, \tilde{\boldsymbol{\theta}}) \leq$

$\log p(\mathbf{d}, \boldsymbol{\theta}|\mathbf{u})$ that touches the objective function at the current estimates, i.e., $Q(\tilde{\mathbf{d}}, \tilde{\boldsymbol{\theta}}|\tilde{\mathbf{d}}, \tilde{\boldsymbol{\theta}}) = \log p(\tilde{\mathbf{d}}, \tilde{\boldsymbol{\theta}}|\mathbf{u})$, and subsequently optimizing this lower bound to find new parameter estimates:

$$(\tilde{\mathbf{d}}, \tilde{\boldsymbol{\theta}}) \leftarrow \arg\max_{(\mathbf{d}, \boldsymbol{\theta})} Q(\mathbf{d}, \boldsymbol{\theta}|\tilde{\mathbf{d}}, \tilde{\boldsymbol{\theta}}). \tag{1}$$

By design, this scheme guarantees that $\log p(\mathbf{d}, \boldsymbol{\theta}|\mathbf{u})$ is increased with every new iteration. The lower bound is constructed using Jensen's inequality, effectively "filling in" the unknown node assignments with their expectations:

$$Q(\mathbf{d}, \boldsymbol{\theta}|\tilde{\mathbf{d}}, \tilde{\boldsymbol{\theta}}) \equiv \sum_{i=1}^{I} \sum_{j=1}^{J} w_{i,j}(\tilde{\mathbf{d}}, \tilde{\boldsymbol{\theta}}) \log\left[\frac{p(u_i|n_i = j, \boldsymbol{\theta})p(n_i = j|\mathbf{d})}{w_{i,j}(\tilde{\mathbf{d}}, \tilde{\boldsymbol{\theta}})}\right] + \log\left[\frac{p(\boldsymbol{\theta})p(\mathbf{d})}{p(\mathbf{u})}\right]$$

$$\leq \sum_{i=1}^{I} \log\underbrace{\left[\sum_{j=1}^{J} \frac{p(u_i|n_i = j, \boldsymbol{\theta})p(n_i = j|\mathbf{d})}{w_{i,j}(\tilde{\mathbf{d}}, \tilde{\boldsymbol{\theta}})} w_{i,j}(\tilde{\mathbf{d}}, \tilde{\boldsymbol{\theta}})\right]}_{p(u_i|\mathbf{d}, \boldsymbol{\theta})} + \log\left[\frac{p(\boldsymbol{\theta})p(\mathbf{d})}{p(\mathbf{u})}\right]$$

$$= \log p(\mathbf{d}, \boldsymbol{\theta}|\mathbf{u}),$$

where

$$w_{i,j}(\mathbf{d}, \boldsymbol{\theta}) = p(n_i = j|u_i, \mathbf{d}, \boldsymbol{\theta}) = \frac{\theta_{v_j, u_i}\beta^b\left(y_j - (x_i + d_i)\right)}{\sum_{j'=1}^{J} \theta_{v_{j'}, u_i}\beta^b\left(y_{j'} - (x_i + d_i)\right)} \tag{2}$$

weighs the association of each voxel i with each of the j nodes, so that $\sum_{j=1}^{J} w_{i,j} = 1, \forall i$. Note that most $w_{i,j} = 0$, due to the limited spatial support of B-splines.

Finding new parameter estimates by solving Eq. (1) readily yields the following closed-form update for $\boldsymbol{\theta}$:

$$\tilde{\theta}_{k,l} \leftarrow \frac{N_{k,l} + (\alpha_0^l - 1)}{\sum_{l'=1}^{L}\left(N_{k,l'} + (\alpha_0^{l'} - 1)\right)} \quad \forall k, l, \tag{3}$$

where

$$N_{k,l} = \sum_{i=1}^{I} \sum_{j=1}^{J} [u_i = l][v_j = k]w_{i,j} \tag{4}$$

can be interpreted as the effective number of voxels with intensity l that were assigned to nodes of class k. The corresponding update for $\mathbf{d}$ is not given in closed form, but an efficient and accurate approximation can be obtained by observing that B-splines rapidly become more Gaussian-like as the order b increases: $\beta^b(z) \simeq \mathcal{N}(z|0, \sigma_b^2)$ for an appropriate choice of variance σ_b^2. Plugging in this approximation yields an objective function that is quadratic in $\mathbf{d}$, and that therefore has a closed-form solution:

$$\tilde{\mathbf{d}} \simeq \arg\min_{\mathbf{d}}\left[\sum_{i=1}^{I} \sum_{j=1}^{J} w_{i,j}\frac{(y_j - x_i - d_i)^2}{\sigma_b^2} + \gamma\mathbf{d}^{\mathsf{T}}\boldsymbol{\Gamma}^{\mathsf{T}}\boldsymbol{\Gamma}\mathbf{d}\right] = \mathbf{S}\boldsymbol{\delta}, \tag{5}$$

where

$$\mathbf{S} = \left(\mathbf{I}_I + \gamma\sigma_b^2\mathbf{\Gamma}^{\mathrm{T}}\mathbf{\Gamma}\right)^{-1}, \quad \boldsymbol{\delta} = (\delta_1,\dots,\delta_I)^{\mathrm{T}}, \quad \delta_i = \sum_{j=1}^{J} w_{i,j}\,y_j - x_i. \quad (6)$$

Thus, in each voxel i a local "vote" for a displacement δ_i is made that would recover the distance between the node(s) the voxel associates with, and its actual position. These local votes are then spatially smoothed by a $I \times I$ matrix $\mathbf{S}$ that implements a shift-invariant low-pass filter, to give the new estimate for $\mathbf{d}$. In summary, the proposed EM optimizer iteratively cycles between updating the expected node assignments $w_{i,j}$ (Eq. (2)) and the estimates of $\boldsymbol{\theta}$ (Eq. (3)) and $\mathbf{d}$ (Eq. (5)). In the Appendix, we show that this optimization scheme effectively performs MI-based registration with partial volume interpolation [18,19].

In our implementation, we initialize the algorithm by setting $\theta_{k,l}^0 = 1/L, \forall k,l$ and $d_i^0 = 0, \forall i$, and we use cubic B-splines ($b = 3$) in order to obtain an accurate Gaussian approximation, where σ_b^2 is set so that $\mathcal{N}(0|0,\sigma_b^2) = \beta^b(0)$. For $\mathbf{\Gamma}$, we use a filter that computes local curvature using finite differences (a so-called bending energy or biharmonic model), and we use $\boldsymbol{\alpha}_0 = 2\cdot 1$. Since the smoothing matrix $\mathbf{S}$ is circulant, the filtering can be performed as element-wise multiplication in the Fourier domain. Implemented in ITK 5.0 and MATLAB 9.6 on an Intel Core i7-5930K computer with Intel MKL's FFTW library, one iteration of the EM algorithm takes around 3.5 s for images of size $256 \times 176 \times 256$.

4   Sampling

Rather than simply obtaining point estimates $(\widehat{\mathbf{d}}, \widehat{\boldsymbol{\theta}})$, the uncertainty of these estimates can be quantified by Monte Carlo sampling from the posterior distribution $p(\mathbf{d}, \boldsymbol{\theta}|\mathbf{u})$. Since $p(\mathbf{d}, \boldsymbol{\theta}|\mathbf{u}) = \sum_{\mathbf{n}} p(\mathbf{d}, \boldsymbol{\theta}, \mathbf{n}|\mathbf{u})$, we can again exploit the latent node assignments $\mathbf{n}$ to obtain an efficient sampling strategy: Starting from an initialization $(\mathbf{d}^{(0)}, \boldsymbol{\theta}^{(0)}) = (\widehat{\mathbf{d}}, \widehat{\boldsymbol{\theta}})$, a Gibbs sampler of $p(\mathbf{d}, \boldsymbol{\theta}, \mathbf{n}|\mathbf{u})$ is obtained by the iterative scheme

$$\mathbf{n}^{(\tau+1)} \sim p(\mathbf{n}|\mathbf{d}^{(\tau)}, \boldsymbol{\theta}^{(\tau)}, \mathbf{u}) = \prod_{i=1}^{I}\prod_{j=1}^{J}\left\{w_{i,j}(\mathbf{d}^{(\tau)}, \boldsymbol{\theta}^{(\tau)})\right\}^{[n_i=j]}$$

$$\boldsymbol{\theta}^{(\tau+1)} \sim p(\boldsymbol{\theta}|\mathbf{u}, \mathbf{n}^{(\tau+1)}) = \prod_{k=1}^{K}\mathrm{Dir}\left(\boldsymbol{\theta}_k|\boldsymbol{\alpha}_k\right), \ \boldsymbol{\alpha}_k = (N_{k,1}^{(\tau+1)},\dots,N_{k,L}^{(\tau+1)})^{\mathrm{T}} + \boldsymbol{\alpha}_0$$

$$\mathbf{d}^{(\tau+1)} \sim p(\mathbf{d}|\mathbf{u}, \mathbf{n}^{(\tau+1)}) = \mathcal{N}\left(\mathbf{d}\,|\,\mathbf{S}\boldsymbol{\delta}^{(\tau+1)}, \sigma_b^2\mathbf{S}\right),$$

where $N_{k,l}^{(\tau+1)}$, and $\boldsymbol{\delta}^{(\tau+1)}$ are as defined in Eqs. (4) and (6) but with hard node assignments $w_{i,j} = [n_i^{(\tau+1)} = j]$. After discarding the first T_0 burn-in sweeps, the set $\{\mathbf{d}^{(\tau)}, \boldsymbol{\theta}^{(\tau)}\}_{\tau=T_0+1}^{T}$ contains $(T - T_0)$ valid samples of the target distribution

$p(\mathbf{d}, \boldsymbol{\theta}|\mathbf{u})$. Since the required computations are very similar to those of the EM algorithm ($\mathbf{d}^{(\tau+1)}$ can again be computed via the Fourier domain), implementing the sampler requires very little additional code, and the computation time of a single sweep is comparable to that of one EM iteration.

As in other work [3–9], the deformation regularization parameter γ can also be inferred automatically, rather than set by the user. When a non-informative gamma distribution $\mathrm{Gam}(\gamma|\alpha_0, \beta_0)$ with shape $\alpha_0 = 1$ and rate $\beta_0 = 0$ is used as a conjugate prior for γ, this can be accomplished by simply including a fourth step in the sampler: $\gamma^{(\tau+1)} \sim p(\gamma|\mathbf{d}^{(\tau+1)}) = \mathrm{Gam}(\frac{I}{2} + 1, \frac{1}{2}\|\mathbf{\Gamma d}^{(\tau+1)}\|^2)$.

5   Experiments

In order to perform an initial, preliminary comparison of the performance of the proposed optimizer with that of the well-known free-form deformation method Elastix (v. 4.8) [13], we co-registered the T2-weighted brain scans of 6 healthy subjects to the T1-weighted scan of 10 other healthy subjects in the OASIS database [20]. We first segmented and bias field corrected each image (including an additional T1w scan for the 6 subjects with T2w) with a whole-brain segmentation tool [21], and affinely pre-registered each of the registration pairs with Elastix. Registration accuracy was quantified by computing the Dice scores between the T1-based segmentations for each of the 60 T2-T1 registration pairs, averaged over the 10 largest brain structures.

For Elastix, we varied the B-spline grid spacing between 4, 3.5, 3, and 2.5 voxels, and the number of iterations per multi-resolution level between 500 (which is the default) and 2000 (which is recommended for best results). For each parameter variation, we used recommended and default settings, with a 4-level multi-resolution strategy and 5000 off-grid samples per iteration. The proposed method used the same multi-resolution regime, and varied the deformation regularization parameter γ between 14.9, 8.7, 4.8 and 2.3 to achieve the same effective number of degrees of freedom (measured as the trace of the smoothing matrix $\mathbf{S}$ [22]) as the corresponding B-spline deformation models in Elastix. The number of iterations per resolution level was also varied, between 25, 50 and 100.

The middle row of Fig. 1 shows an example registration obtained with the proposed method when the maximum degrees of freedom and 100 iterations are used. The top row shows quantitative results for the proposed method across the various settings, along with the corresponding results obtained with Elastix. It can be seen that the computational burden (left plot) of the proposed method is independent of the flexibility of the deformation models, whereas for Elastix the computation time increases sharply as more degrees of freedom are added. Furthermore, whereas it is possible to obtain better Dice scores for both algorithms by increasing the number of iterations and the degrees of freedom (middle plot), the proposed method does so more effectively, reaching higher average accuracy levels in 2.5 min (25 iterations at the highest flexibility), than the best achievable performance of Elastix, taking around 23 min (2000 iterations at B-spline spacing of 3 voxels). Finally, we also show the percentage of voxels with a Jacobian determinant lower or equal to zero for both methods (right plot), indicating that the proposed method's deformation model is better behaved.

The bottom row and the last image on the middle row of Fig. 1 illustrate the proposed sampler (initialized by the optimizer with $\gamma = 2.3$) across 4000 samples after a burn-in of 1000 sweeps, where γ was kept constant for the first 100 sweeps. The uncertainty (last image, middle row) is shown as the standard deviation (measured in voxels) in each of the three spatial directions, and is encoded as red for superior-inferior, blue for left-right, and green for anterior-posterior. The bottom row shows the estimated posterior distribution of γ, and two deformation field samples (also including superior-inferior), zoomed-in on a region of interest and color-coded according to displacement magnitude.

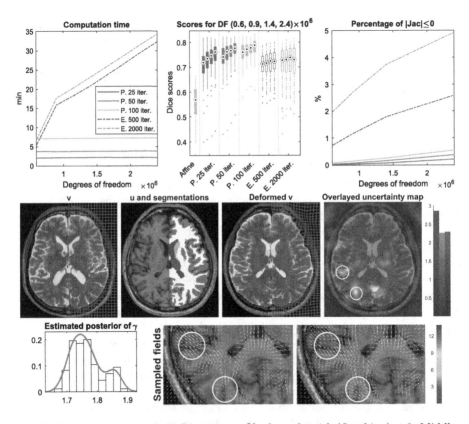

Fig. 1. Top: computation time; Dice scores; % of voxels with $|$Jacobian$| \leq 0$. Middle: $\mathbf{v}$; $\mathbf{u}$ with segmentations partially overlayed; deformed $\mathbf{v}$; uncertainty map. Bottom: posterior of γ; two deformation field samples.   P = Proposed method, E = Elastix.

6   Discussion

In this paper we have proposed a probabilistic model that directly incorporates the MI metric into a demons-like optimization scheme. We have shown that the resulting algorithm can potentially be more accurate and significantly faster than the free-form deformation method implemented in Elastix. We have also demonstrated that a Monte Carlo sampler, using largely the same code base, can directly produce uncertainty estimates in MI-based registration – to the best of our knowledge the first method in the literature to do so.

We note that although the generative model encodes MI in this paper, it can be used for a wide range of predictive distributions, including the Gaussian noise assumption underlying the SSD criterion. Although not reported here, preliminary experiments indicate that the proposed optimizer achieves comparable registration accuracies to the original demons algorithm [2] in this setting. The proposed sampler directly endows the demons algorithm with the first method to assess the uncertainty in its nonparametric deformation fields, the effective number of degrees of freedom of which is in the millions (compared to mere thousands in existing work for uncertainty estimation in registration [3–10]).

Given the close similarity between the two methods, in future work we plan to investigate whether the same update modification that makes the demons algorithm diffeomorphic [2] can also be used with the proposed optimizer.

Acknowledgments. This project has received funding from the European Union's Horizon 2020 research and innovation programme under the Marie Skło-dowska-Curie grant agreement No 765148; the Danish Council for Independent Research under grant number DFF611100291; and the NIH National Institute on Aging under grant number R21AG050122.

Appendix: Connection with MI-based registration

MI-based registration with partial volume interpolation can be interpreted as implicitly using the proposed generative model but with a different optimization strategy, in which EM is used to estimate $\boldsymbol{\theta}$ but not $\mathbf{d}$. In particular, $\widehat{\mathbf{d}}$ can also be estimated by optimizing $\log p(\mathbf{d}, \widehat{\boldsymbol{\theta}}_d|\mathbf{u})$ for $\mathbf{d}$ with a general-purpose optimizer, where $\widehat{\boldsymbol{\theta}}_d = \arg\max_\theta \log p(\mathbf{d}, \boldsymbol{\theta}|\mathbf{u})$ involves an inner optimization that for each $\mathbf{d}$ estimates a matched $\widehat{\boldsymbol{\theta}}_d$ de novo from starting values $\theta^0_{k,l} = 1/L, \forall k, l$ by interleaving the EM Eqs. (2) and (3). When a flat prior $p(\boldsymbol{\theta}) \propto 1$ is used, the resulting effective registration criterion is then directly related to MI as follows:

$$\log p(\mathbf{d}, \widehat{\boldsymbol{\theta}}_d|\mathbf{u}) \simeq I\mathrm{MI}(\mathbf{d}) + \log p(\mathbf{d}) + \mathrm{const}, \tag{7}$$

where

$$\mathrm{MI}(\mathbf{d}) = \sum_{k=1}^{K}\sum_{l=1}^{L} n_{k,l} \log \frac{n_{k,l}}{n_k \, n_l} \quad \text{with} \quad n_{k,l} = \frac{N_{k,l}}{I}, \ n_k = \sum_l n_{k,l}, \ n_l = \sum_k n_{k,l}$$

is the MI criterion using partial volume interpolation [18,19], in which joint histogram counts $N_{k,l}$ are computed from fractional weights $\bar{w}_{i,j}^d = \beta^b(y_j - (x_i + d_i))$ as in Eq. (4). To see why Eq. (7) holds, we can also write MI($\mathbf{d}$) as

$$\text{MI}(\mathbf{d}) = \frac{1}{I} \sum_{i=1}^{I} \sum_{j=1}^{J} \bar{w}_{i,j}^d \log \bar{\theta}_{v_j,u_i}^d - \underbrace{\sum_{l=1}^{L} n_l \log n_l}_{\text{const}} \quad \text{with} \quad \bar{\theta}_{kl}^d = n_{k,l}/n_k, \quad (8)$$

and, since $\log p(\mathbf{d}, \widehat{\boldsymbol{\theta}}_d) = Q(\mathbf{d}, \widehat{\boldsymbol{\theta}}_d | \mathbf{d}, \widehat{\boldsymbol{\theta}}_d)$,

$$\log p(\mathbf{d}, \widehat{\boldsymbol{\theta}}_d | \mathbf{u}) - \log p(\mathbf{d}) = \sum_{i=1}^{I} \sum_{j=1}^{J} \widehat{w}_{i,j}^d \log \widehat{\theta}_{v_j,u_i}^d$$
$$- \sum_i D_{KL} \left[p(n_i | u_i, \mathbf{d}, \widehat{\boldsymbol{\theta}}_d) \, \| \, p(n_i | \mathbf{d}) \right] + \text{const}, \quad (9)$$

where $\widehat{w}_{i,j}^d = w_{i,j}(\mathbf{d}, \widehat{\boldsymbol{\theta}}_d)$ and $D_{KL}(.\|.)$ denotes the Kullback-Leibler (KL) divergence. Comparing Eqs. (8) and (9), and noting that $\bar{w}_{i,j}^d$ and $\bar{\boldsymbol{\theta}}_d$ are precisely the weights and estimate of $\boldsymbol{\theta}$ in the first iteration of the inner EM optimization, MI-based registration can therefore be interpreted as making a "lazy" attempt at measuring $\log p(\mathbf{d}, \widehat{\boldsymbol{\theta}}_d)$, using only a single iteration in the inner optimization of $\widehat{\boldsymbol{\theta}}_d$, and ignoring the KL divergence between the prior and the posterior node assignment distributions. In the special case where $p(n_i | \mathbf{d})$ takes only binary values $\{0, 1\}$, the approximation in Eq. (7) will be exact since the EM algorithm then immediately finds $\widehat{\boldsymbol{\theta}}_d$ in its first iteration and the KL divergence term vanishes. This will happen when B-splines of order $b = 0$ are used, or for first-order B-splines ($b = 1$) whenever the image grids of $\mathbf{u}$ and $\mathbf{v}$ perfectly align.

References

1. Thirion, J.P.: Image matching as a diffusion process: an analogy with Maxwell's demons. Med. Image Anal. **2**(3), 243–260 (1998)
2. Vercauteren, T., Pennec, X., Perchant, A., Ayache, N.: Diffeomorphic demons: efficient non-parametric image registration. NeuroImage **45**(1), S61–S72 (2009)
3. Simpson, I.J., Schnabel, J.A., Groves, A.R., Andersson, J.L., Woolrich, M.W.: Probabilistic inference of regularisation in non-rigid registration. NeuroImage **59**(3), 2438–2451 (2012)
4. Simpson, I.J.A., et al.: A bayesian approach for spatially adaptive regularisation in non-rigid registration. In: Mori, K., Sakuma, I., Sato, Y., Barillot, C., Navab, N. (eds.) MICCAI 2013. LNCS, vol. 8150, pp. 10–18. Springer, Heidelberg (2013). https://doi.org/10.1007/978-3-642-40763-5_2
5. Simpson, I.J., et al.: Probabilistic non-linear registration with spatially adaptive regularisation. Med. Image Anal. **26**(1), 203–216 (2015)
6. Le Folgoc, L., Delingette, H., Criminisi, A., Ayache, N.: Sparse bayesian registration of medical images for self-tuning of parameters and spatially adaptive parametrization of displacements. Med. Image Anal. **36**, 79–97 (2017)

7. Risholm, P., Samset, E., Wells, W.: Bayesian estimation of deformation and elastic parameters in non-rigid registration. In: Fischer, B., Dawant, B.M., Lorenz, C. (eds.) WBIR 2010. LNCS, vol. 6204, pp. 104–115. Springer, Heidelberg (2010). https://doi.org/10.1007/978-3-642-14366-3_10
8. Risholm, P., Janoos, F., Norton, I., Golby, A.J., Wells III, W.M.: Bayesian characterization of uncertainty in intra-subject non-rigid registration. Med. Image Anal. **17**(5), 538–555 (2013)
9. Le Folgoc, L., Delingette, H., Criminisi, A., Ayache, N.: Quantifying registration uncertainty with sparse bayesian modelling. IEEE Trans. Med. Imaging **36**(2), 607–617 (2016)
10. Pursley, J., et al.: A Bayesian nonrigid registration method to enhance intraoperative target definition in image-guided prostate procedures through uncertainty characterization. Med. Phys. **39**(11), 6858–6867 (2012)
11. Rueckert, D., Sonoda, L.I., Hayes, C., Hill, D.L., Leach, M.O., Hawkes, D.J.: Nonrigid registration using free-form deformations: application to breast MR images. IEEE Trans. Med. Imaging **18**(8), 712–721 (1999)
12. Modat, M., et al.: Fast free-form deformation using graphics processing units. Comput. Methods Prog. Biomed. **98**(3), 278–284 (2010)
13. Klein, S., Staring, M., Murphy, K., Viergever, M.A., Pluim, J.P.: Elastix: a toolbox for intensity-based medical image registration. IEEE Trans. Med. Imaging **29**(1), 196–205 (2010)
14. Modat, M., Vercauteren, T., Ridgway, G.R., Hawkes, D.J., Fox, N.C., Ourselin, S.: Diffeomorphic demons using normalized mutual information, evaluation on multi-modal brain MR images. In: SPIE Medical Imaging 2010: Image Processing, vol. 7623, p. 76232K (2010)
15. Lu, H., et al.: Multi-modal diffeomorphic demons registration based on point-wise mutual information. In: 2010 IEEE International Symposium on Biomedical Imaging: From Nano to Macro, pp. 372–375 (2010)
16. Risser, L., Heinrich, M.P., Rueckert, D., Schnabel, J.A.: Multi-modal diffeomorphic registration using mutual information: application to the registration of CT and MR pulmonary images. In: Proceedings MICCAI Workshop PIA (2011)
17. Janoos, F., Risholm, P., Wells, W.: Bayesian characterization of uncertainty in multi-modal image registration. In: Dawant, B.M., Christensen, G.E., Fitzpatrick, J.M., Rueckert, D. (eds.) WBIR 2012. LNCS, vol. 7359, pp. 50–59. Springer, Heidelberg (2012). https://doi.org/10.1007/978-3-642-31340-0_6
18. Maes, F., Collignon, A., Vandermeulen, D., Marchal, G., Suetens, P.: Multimodality image registration by maximization of mutual information. IEEE Trans. Med. Imaging **16**(2), 187–198 (1997)
19. Chen, H.M., Varshney, P.K.: Mutual information-based CT-MR brain image registration using generalized partial volume joint histogram estimation. IEEE Trans. Med. Imaging **22**(9), 1111–1119 (2003)
20. Marcus, D.S., Wang, T.H., Parker, J., Csernansky, J.G., Morris, J.C., Buckner, R.L.: Open access series of imaging studies (OASIS): cross-sectional MRI data in young, middle aged, nondemented, and demented older adults. J. Cogn. Neurosci. **19**(9), 1498–1507 (2007)
21. Puonti, O., Iglesias, J.E., Van Leemput, K.: Fast and sequence-adaptive whole-brain segmentation using parametric bayesian modeling. NeuroImage **143**, 235–249 (2016)
22. Hastie, T., Tibshirani, R., Friedman, J.: The Elements of Statistical Learning. Springer Series in Statistics, 2nd edn. Springer, New York (2009). https://doi.org/10.1007/978-0-387-84858-7

Quantifying Uncertainty of Deep Neural Networks in Skin Lesion Classification

Pieter Van Molle[1(✉)], Tim Verbelen[1], Cedric De Boom[1], Bert Vankeirsbilck[1], Jonas De Vylder[2], Bart Diricx[2], Tom Kimpe[2], Pieter Simoens[1], and Bart Dhoedt[1]

[1] IDLab, Department of Information Technology at Ghent University - imec, Ghent, Belgium
{pieter.vanmolle,tim.verbelen,cedric.deboom,bert.vankeirsbilck, pieter.simoens,bart.dhoedt}@ugent.be
[2] Barco N.V., Kortrijk, Belgium
{jonas.devylder,bart.diricx,tom.kimpe}@barco.com

Abstract. Deep neural networks are becoming the new standard for automated image classification and segmentation. Recently, such models are also gaining traction in the context of medical diagnosis. However, when using a neural network as a decision support tool, it is important to also quantify the (un)certainty regarding the outputs of the system. Current Bayesian techniques approximate the true predictive output distribution via sampling, and quantify the uncertainty based on the variance of the output samples. In this paper, we highlight the limitations of a variance based metric, and propose a novel uncertainty metric based on the overlap of the output distributions. We show that this yields promising results on the HAM10000 dataset for skin lesion classification.

Keywords: Deep learning · Uncertainty · Dermatology · Skin lesions

1 Introduction

Since the rise of deep learning [10], deep neural network architectures have continued to set new state-of-the-art benchmarks for a variety of computer vision tasks, such as large-scale image classification [8,22,24], object localization [5,6,18], and semantic segmentation [15,19]. Because of these successes, deep learning also gained more traction in medicine [12,14,21,23], and in particular in skin lesion classification using dermoscopic images [3]. However, care has to be taken when employing deep neural networks to support medical diagnosis. It is known that neural networks are only a point estimate of the true underlying distribution, and the softmax output layer that is used to get a probability score is typically "over-confident" for one class [4]. This is especially the case for unbalanced datasets, where one class is over-sampled a lot, which is quite common in medical datasets. For example, in the case of skin lesion classification, datasets typically contain many more benign lesions compared to malignant ones.

© Springer Nature Switzerland AG 2019
H. Greenspan et al. (Eds.): CLIP 2019/UNSURE 2019, LNCS 11840, pp. 52–61, 2019.
https://doi.org/10.1007/978-3-030-32689-0_6

Hence, correctly capturing output uncertainty is indispensable when offering a deep learning algorithm to a dermatologist as a decision support tool. Providing information on the uncertainty of the output is even more important when these algorithms are used in a pre-screening phase by the general practitioners, or by patients for self-diagnosis.

Bayesian modelling offers a set of mathematically sound tools to reason about uncertainty, by providing a probability density over the outcomes given the data. Despite some recent advances in fitting deep learning in the Bayesian framework [2,7], Bayesian neural networks have not seen a high adoption rate, mainly because of difficulties in implementation and excessive training times. In [4], the authors prove that training a neural network with dropout approximates variational inference. Obtaining an output distribution estimate then boils down to Monte Carlo (MC) sampling the prediction, while leaving dropout enabled.

In order to quantify the output uncertainty, the most common metric used is the variance of the different output samples, i.e. the predictive variance. However, we argue that this metric falls short to be used in a decision support tool. First, this metric yields hard to interpret quantities, typically very small in absolute value. Second, the predictive variance does not take into account any overlap of the output distributions for the different classes, which can indicate class confusion. In this paper, we propose a novel uncertainty metric that has a sound range between 0 (very certain) and 1 (not certain at all) and is therefore easy to interpret. Our metric also takes into account distribution overlap between the different output classes. We apply our metric on the case of skin lesion classification, using the HAM10000 dataset [25]. We show that indeed the model yields a much higher accuracy on the fraction of the test set where the uncertainty is low. Additionally, we observe that the model is most confident on the class with most training data.

In the next section we first introduce the Bayesian framework and how neural networks can be used to approximate the true posterior distribution. In Sect. 3 we then present our metric for quantifying uncertainty on the neural network output. In Sect. 4 we evaluate our metric on a skin lesion classification task using the HAM10000 dataset. Finally we discuss our results and conclude with some pointers to future work.

2   Bayesian Neural Networks

A neural network can be considered a probabilistic model $p(y|x, w)$, where, given an input $x \in \mathbb{R}^d$, a probability is assigned to each of the possible outputs $y \in \mathcal{Y}$, using the parameters of the network w. In case of classification, $\mathcal{Y}$ is the set of labels, and $p(y|x, w)$ is a softmax distribution over these labels. Given a dataset $\mathcal{D}$ of samples (x_i, y_i), the optimal set of parameters $w^\star$ can be learned using maximum likelihood estimation (MLE):

$$w^\star = \arg\max_w \log p(\mathcal{D}|w)$$

$$= \arg\max_w \sum_i \log p(y_i|x_i, w).$$

To cast a neural network as a Bayesian model, the weights are no longer fixed values, but rather randomly drawn from a prior distribution $p(w)$. By observing data, new insight into the weights can be gained, resulting in the posterior $p(w|\mathcal{D})$. Using the posterior, a predictive distribution over the outputs y^* can be calculated for an unseen data point x^*, by marginalizing over all possible values for the weights:

$$p(y^*|x^*, \mathcal{D}) = \int p(y^*|x^*, w)p(w|\mathcal{D})dw,$$

where, following Bayes' theorem,

$$p(w|\mathcal{D}) = \frac{p(\mathcal{D}|w)p(w)}{p(\mathcal{D})}$$

$$= \frac{p(\mathcal{D}|w)p(w)}{\int p(\mathcal{D}|w)p(w)dw}.$$

Unfortunately, this value cannot be calculated analytically, due to the intractable integral in the denominator. Variational inference addresses this issue, by approximating the true posterior $p(w|\mathcal{D})$ with a parameterized distribution $q_\theta(w)$, which closely resembles the true posterior. The optimal parameters θ^* for this distribution can be found by minimizing the Kullback-Leibler (KL) divergence with the true posterior on the weights:

$$\theta^* = \arg\max_\theta \mathrm{KL}\left[q_\theta(w)||p(w|\mathcal{D})\right]$$

$$= \arg\max_\theta \int q_\theta(w) \log \frac{q_\theta(w)}{p(w)p(\mathcal{D}|w)}dw,$$

which is equivalent to minimizing the expected lower bound (ELBO) given by

$$\mathrm{KL}\left[q_\theta(w)||p(w)\right] - \mathbb{E}_q[\log p(\mathcal{D}|w)].$$

In [4], the authors relate dropout training of a neural network to variational inference, by approximating the true posterior $p(w|\mathcal{D})$ with $q(w)$, where sampling weights $w \sim q(w)$ is equivalent to performing dropout on the network. The resulting predictive distribution then becomes

$$q(y^*|x^*) = \int p(y^*|x^*, w)q(w)dw. \tag{1}$$

Given the predictive distribution in (1), an unbiased estimator can be obtained using Monte Carlo sampling:

$$\hat{q}(y^*|x^*) = \frac{1}{T} \sum_{t=1}^{T} p(y^*|x^*, \hat{w}_t), \tag{2}$$

where the parameters of the network $\hat{w}_t$ are drawn from the dropout distribution, for a pre-defined number of times T.

3   Quantifying Output Uncertainty

Quantifying output uncertainty of an (approximate) Bayesian neural network is typically done using the predictive variance [11], i.e. the variance of the outputs of the predictive distribution:

$$\text{Var}_{\hat{q}_\theta(y^*|x^*)}(y^*) = \mathbb{E}_{\hat{q}_\theta(y^*|x^*)}[y^{*\otimes 2}] - \mathbb{E}_{\hat{q}_\theta(y^*|x^*)}[y^*]^{\otimes 2}.$$

In a medical context, this has been applied for both detection tasks [13,17], as well as segmentation tasks [11,16,20,26].

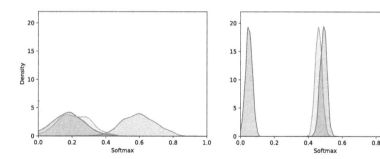

Fig. 1. The true per-class output probability densities for two examples in a three-way classification problem. Although the predictive variance is high in the left example and low in the right example, intuitively one would asses that the model is more certain that "green" is the correct label for the left example. (Color figure online)

However, the predictive variance typically has a small value range, which is hard to interpret for a medical professional. Moreover, this fails to capture the uncertainty of the model on its top-1 classification, which is often of most importance for decision support. Consider the following intuitive example. A Bayesian neural network is trained on a three-way classification problem. Figure 1 shows two examples of a predictive distribution for each class. Although both examples would get assigned the label "green", there is a lot to say about the corresponding uncertainty. By inspecting the densities for the first example, on the left, we would argue that the "green" class is most likely the ground truth class, since there is almost no overlap between the "green" density and the others. The second example, on the right, has highly overlapping densities for the "green" and the "orange" class. Therefore, we cannot say for sure that the "green" class is the ground truth class.

Contradictory to this intuition, using the predictive variance as uncertainty metric, a high uncertainty would be assigned to the first example, and a low uncertainty to the second example. Therefore, we propose a novel metric, that is based on the overlap between distributions, rather than their variance. In a first step, we approximate the output distributions using the estimator in (2), obtaining a sample distribution of T output values for each class. In a second step, we select only those distributions d_1 and d_2 for the top-2 classes, having the highest and second to highest mean. Finally, we estimate the overlap between these distributions using the normalized Bhattacharyya coefficient [1]. For this, we construct a histogram h_1 for d_1, and a histogram h_2 for d_2, both with n bins. The normalized Bhattacharyya coefficient is then given by:

$$BC(h_1, h_2) = \frac{1}{n} \sum_{i=1}^{n} \sqrt{h_{1_i} h_{2_i}}$$

in which h_{1_i} and h_{2_i} are the bin sizes for the i-th bin of respective histograms h_1 and h_2. The result is a value between 0 and 1, where 0 indicates no overlap between distributions, while 1 indicates a perfect overlap (i.e. the distributions are identical). We now interpret this value as a measure for the output uncertainty, where a high and a low value respectively indicate a high and a low uncertainty. We refer to this value as the *BC uncertainty*. An example of how to calculate the BC uncertainty, given a dropout neural network, is shown in Fig. 2.

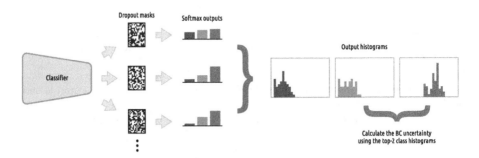

Fig. 2. An overview of how to calculate the BC uncertainty for a given example, for the case of a neural network trained with dropout. The example is passed T times through the network. At each pass, a different dropout mask is sampled from the dropout distribution, resulting in T softmax outputs. From these outputs, we construct a histogram for the top-2 classes, having the highest and second to highest mean. Using these histograms, we calculate the BC uncertainty.

4   Experiments

We apply our method to the problem of skin lesion classification, using the HAM10000 dataset [25]. This dataset contains 10,015 dermoscopic images of common pigmented skin lesions, divided over seven classes. Similar to other medical datasets, this dataset is heavily imbalanced. The images are down-scaled to 224×224 pixels, and normalized. We randomly split the full dataset into a training set (9,013 images, approximately 90%), a validation set, and a hold-out test set (both 501 images, approximately 5%). We use the training and validation set to train a deep neural network architecture and optimize hyperparameters.

Given the limited amount of training data available, we use a ResNet50 network [8], which was pre-trained on ImageNet [10], as a feature extractor. We fix the parameters of the network, and replace the final layer with our own head for classification. The head consists of two fully connected hidden layers, respectively having 512 and 64 units, followed by a fully connected output layer with 7 units. Both hidden layers have rectified linear unit (ReLU) activations. We apply dropout after every hidden layer, with a dropout probability of 0.6. We augment the training set by randomly flipping the images, both horizontally and vertically, with a probability of 0.5. We train the network for 64 epochs, using a batch size of 128. The trainable parameters are optimized using the Adam [9] optimizer, with an initial learning rate of 0.0001, and an exponential decay rate for the first and second order momentum of respectively 0.9 and 0.999.

We obtain predictions, as well as BC uncertainties, for the hold-out test set, by means of MC sampling, with $T = 100$, achieving an accuracy of 0.82. To calculate the BC uncertainty for each image, we partition the output values into histograms with 100 bins ($n = 100$).

4.1   Uncertainty vs Accuracy

We evaluate the BC uncertainty for each image in the test set, and plot the accuracy when grouping test set images according to their BC uncertainty in Fig. 3. More than half of the images (268 out of 501) are classified with very low uncertainty (BC = 0.0), with a resulting accuracy of 0.95. The higher the BC uncertainty, the lower the accuracy becomes. This indicates that, indeed, our metric yields better classification accuracy for lower uncertainty, and vice versa.

4.2   The (un)certain Cases

In Fig. 4, we show four example images from the dataset, with their respective output histograms for each class. The top-2 classes, which are used to calculate the BC uncertainty, are coloured green and orange, respectively. The first two examples have a high overlap between the top-2 output histograms, and are marked as uncertain. The bottom two have a BC uncertainty of 0, and are clear examples of nevi. All four examples have a similar, small predictive variance. Based on these values, no distinction between uncertainties can be made.

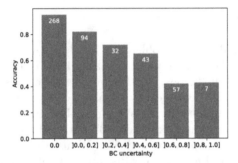

Fig. 3. The accuracy when grouping the test set images according to their BC uncertainty. The special case where the uncertainty is equal to 0.0 is a separate group. For the remainder of the groups, the labels on the X-axis specify the range. The amount of images (out of 501) for each group is specified inside the bar.

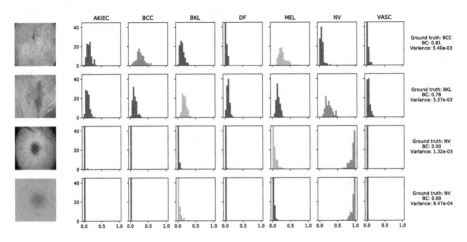

Fig. 4. Examples of skin lesions, and their corresponding output histograms, as well as the BC uncertainty, and the predictive variance, for completeness. The two images at the top have a high uncertainty, while those at the bottom have a low uncertainty. The histograms with the highest and second to highest mean are colored green and orange, respectively. (Color figure online)

4.3   The (un)certain Classes

Finally, Fig. 5 shows the BC uncertainty distributions on a per-class basis. The model is especially confident on the nevi (NV) class. This is to be expected as the HAM10000 contains a large fraction of nevi (67%). This shows that the model is apparently most certain on the class of which it encountered the most examples during training. This indicates the importance of collecting large amounts of data to train a classifier, and of making sure that all classes are sufficiently represented in the train set. However, more research is required to investigate the link between class uncertainty and class imbalance.

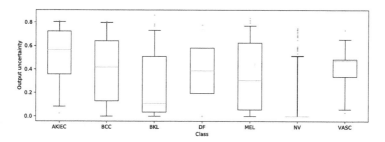

Fig. 5. Distribution of the output uncertainty, for each of the seven classes in the test set. The whiskers represent the 5% and 95% interval. The transparent dots are values outside of this interval.

5   Conclusion

In this work, we present a novel metric to quantify the output uncertainty of a Bayesian neural network. In contrast to existing metrics, which are usually based on the variance of the output samples, our metric estimates the overlap between output distributions. We provide an intuitive example as to why this is preferred. In addition, our metric is bounded between 0 and 1, which makes it easier to interpret.

We evaluate our metric on the problem of skin lesion classification, using the HAM10000 dataset. As is common in medical datasets, this dataset is heavily imbalanced. We illustrate that, indeed, the model is much more accurate on the outputs with low uncertainty, and that, on average, the model is more certain on the class for which it received the most training examples.

Using our metric, we can also extract the images from the dataset the model is most or least certain about. An interesting direction for future work is to check with dermatology experts whether or not these cases match with their own feeling of certainty. The uncertainty metric could also be used in an active learning scenario, where special care is taken to include uncertain examples more often in the train set, to improve the model.

Acknowledgements. Part of this work has been supported by Flanders Innovation & Entrepreneurship, by way of grant agreement HBC.2016.0436/HBC.2018.2028 (DermScan).

References

1. Bhattacharyya, A.: On a measure of divergence between two statistical populations defined by their probability distributions. Bull. Calcutta Math. Soc. **35**, 99–109 (1943)
2. Blundell, C., Cornebise, J., Kavukcuoglu, K., Wierstra, D.: Weight uncertainty in neural networks. arXiv preprint arXiv:1505.05424 (2015)
3. Esteva, A., et al.: Dermatologist-level classification of skin cancer with deep neural networks. Nature **542**, January 2017. http://dx.doi.org/10.1038/nature21056

4. Gal, Y., Ghahramani, Z.: Dropout as a Bayesian approximation: representing model uncertainty in deep learning. In: International Conference on Machine Learning, pp. 1050–1059 (2016)
5. Girshick, R.: Fast R-CNN. In: Proceedings of the IEEE International Conference on Computer Vision, pp. 1440–1448 (2015)
6. Girshick, R., Donahue, J., Darrell, T., Malik, J.: Rich feature hierarchies for accurate object detection and semantic segmentation. In: Proceedings of the IEEE Conference on Computer Vision and Pattern Recognition, pp. 580–587 (2014)
7. Graves, A.: Practical variational inference for neural networks. In: Advances in Neural Information Processing Systems, pp. 2348–2356 (2011)
8. He, K., Zhang, X., Ren, S., Sun, J.: Deep residual learning for image recognition. In: Proceedings of the IEEE Conference on Computer Vision and Pattern Recognition, pp. 770–778 (2016)
9. Kingma, D.P., Ba, J.: Adam: a method for stochastic optimization. arXiv preprint arXiv:1412.6980 (2014)
10. Krizhevsky, A., Sutskever, I., Hinton, G.E.: Imagenet classification with deep convolutional neural networks. In: Advances in Neural Information Processing Systems, pp. 1097–1105 (2012)
11. Kwon, Y., Won, J.H., Kim, B.J., Paik, M.C.: Uncertainty quantification using bayesian neural networks in classification: application to ischemic stroke lesion segmentation (2018)
12. Lee, J.G., et al.: Deep learning in medical imaging: general overview. Korean J. Radiol. **18**(4), 570–584 (2017)
13. Leibig, C., Allken, V., Ayhan, M.S., Berens, P., Wahl, S.: Leveraging uncertainty information from deep neural networks for disease detection. Sci. Rep. **7**(1), 17816 (2017)
14. Litjens, G., et al.: A survey on deep learning in medical image analysis. Med. Image Anal. **42**, 60–88 (2017)
15. Long, J., Shelhamer, E., Darrell, T.: Fully convolutional networks for semantic segmentation. In: Proceedings of the IEEE Conference on Computer Vision and Pattern Recognition, pp. 3431–3440 (2015)
16. Nair, T., Precup, D., Arnold, D.L., Arbel, T.: Exploring uncertainty measures in deep networks for multiple sclerosis lesion detection and segmentation. In: Frangi, A.F., Schnabel, J.A., Davatzikos, C., Alberola-López, C., Fichtinger, G. (eds.) MICCAI 2018. LNCS, vol. 11070, pp. 655–663. Springer, Cham (2018). https://doi.org/10.1007/978-3-030-00928-1_74
17. Ozdemir, O., Woodward, B., Berlin, A.A.: Propagating uncertainty in multi-stage bayesian convolutional neural networks with application to pulmonary nodule detection. arXiv preprint arXiv:1712.00497 (2017)
18. Ren, S., He, K., Girshick, R., Sun, J.: Faster R-CNN: towards real-time object detection with region proposal networks. In: Advances in Neural Information Processing Systems, pp. 91–99 (2015)
19. Ronneberger, O., Fischer, P., Brox, T.: U-Net: convolutional networks for biomedical image segmentation. In: Navab, N., Hornegger, J., Wells, W.M., Frangi, A.F. (eds.) MICCAI 2015. LNCS, vol. 9351, pp. 234–241. Springer, Cham (2015). https://doi.org/10.1007/978-3-319-24574-4_28
20. Seebock, P., et al.: Exploiting epistemic uncertainty of anatomy segmentation for anomaly detection in retinal OCT. IEEE Trans. Med. Imaging (2019)
21. Shen, D., Wu, G., Suk, H.I.: Deep learning in medical image analysis. Annu. Rev. Biomed. Eng. **19**, 221–248 (2017)

22. Simonyan, K., Zisserman, A.: Very deep convolutional networks for large-scale image recognition. arXiv preprint arXiv:1409.1556 (2014)
23. Suzuki, K.: Overview of deep learning in medical imaging. Radiol. Phys. Technol. **10**(3), 257–273 (2017)
24. Szegedy, C., et al.: Going deeper with convolutions. In: Proceedings of the IEEE Conference on Computer Vision and Pattern Recognition, pp. 1–9 (2015)
25. Tschandl, P., Rosendahl, C., Kittler, H.: The ham10000 dataset, a large collection of multi-source dermatoscopic images of common pigmented skin lesions. Sci. data **5**, 180161 (2018)
26. Wang, G., Li, W., Aertsen, M., Deprest, J., Ourselin, S., Vercauteren, T.: Aleatoric uncertainty estimation with test-time augmentation for medical image segmentation with convolutional neural networks. Neurocomputing **338**, 34–45 (2019)

UNSURE 2019: Domain Shift Robustness

A Generalized Approach to Determine Confident Samples for Deep Neural Networks on Unseen Data

Min Zhang[1(✉)], Kevin H. Leung[1,2], Zili Ma[1], Jin Wen[1],
and Gopal Avinash[1]

[1] GE Healthcare, San Ramon, CA 94583, USA
chinazm@gmail.com
[2] The Johns Hopkins University School of Medicine, Baltimore,
MD 21205, USA

Abstract. Deep neural network (DNN) models are widely applied in biomedical image studies since DNN models take advantage of massive data to provide improved performance over traditional machine learning models. However, like any other data-driven models, DNN models still face generalization limitations. For example, a model trained on clinical data from one hospital may not perform as well on data from another hospital. In this work, a novel approach is proposed to determine confident samples from unseen data on which a DNN model will have improved performance. Confident samples are defined as inliers identified by an outlier detector, which is based on projection of training data onto a standard feature space (e.g. ImageNet feature space). The hypothesis of the proposed method is that in a standard feature space, a DNN model will perform better on the inlier data samples and more poorly on the outliers. While projecting the unseen data to a standard feature space, if data points are detected as inliers, then the model will likely have consistent performance on those inliers as those patterns have already been "seen" from the training dataset. To validate our hypothesis, experiments were conducted using publicly available digit image datasets and chest X-ray images from three unseen datasets collected across U.S. and Canada hospitals. The experimental results showed consistently improved performance across various DNN models on all confident samples from unseen datasets.

Keywords: Deep neural network · Feature extraction · Outlier detection · Confident samples

1 Introduction

Deep neural network (DNN) methods have been successfully applied in healthcare domain in recent years. With significant advances in improving the performance of DNN models, it is also crucial to find or detect whether the model has produced a

Electronic supplementary material The online version of this chapter (https://doi.org/10.1007/978-3-030-32689-0_7) contains supplementary material, which is available to authorized users.

H. Greenspan et al. (Eds.): CLIP 2019/UNSURE 2019, LNCS 11840, pp. 65–74, 2019.
https://doi.org/10.1007/978-3-030-32689-0_7

confident prediction, especially for unseen data. The lack of confidence in model predictions may result in poor clinical decisions, which is especially relevant in the medical diagnosis field [1].

In the literature, researchers have estimated the model confidence by quantifying the uncertainty of the model using Monte Carlo dropout [2]. This approach can be applied to image segmentation as in [3] where overall segmentation accuracy improved when pixels with high uncertainty were dropped. Bayesian dropout was also used to estimate prediction uncertainty in diagnosing diabetic retinopathy using fundus images [4]. Diagnostic performance was improved when estimates of uncertainty were used to filter out samples [4].

Other recent work on classification using a filtering strategy for DNNs has been done to filter out instances where the base model prediction is not confident [5]. This method used the outputs of model softmax layer to determine a threshold to optimize sensitivity while preserving precision at a given confidence level [5]. Hendrycks et al. [6] reported a method to measure the confidence score of unseen examples by finding the difference between output probabilities from the final softmax activation layer and true probabilities. In the study, they performed outlier detection between popular computer vision datasets, such as MNIST. However, the out-of-domain examples are visually very different from the in-domain examples in their study. In real world applications, image data from different data sources are often visually indistinguishable. As shown in Fig. 1, the hospital of origin cannot be determined by visual assessment of examples of chest X-ray images from different datasets used in the present study.

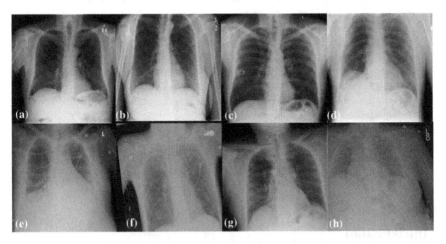

Fig. 1. Good and bad lung field data collected from different data sources. (a) NIH good lung field image, (b) NIH bad lung field image, (c) Source 1 good lung field image, (d) Source 1 bad lung field image, (e) Source 2 good lung field image, (f) Source 2 bad lung field image, (g) Source 3 good lung field image and (h) Source 3 bad lung field image.

In this paper, we propose a generalized novel approach to find the confident predictions when applying DNN models. Borrowing the ideas from Inception Score (IS) [7] and Fréchet Inception Distance (FID) [8] to measure similarity across image datasets, the proposed method projects correctly predicted training data samples onto a standard feature space (ImageNet [9] feature space based on the VGG16 [10] network). An outlier detection model is then trained and built based on a standard feature space to identify the inlier samples on the training dataset. Such inlier samples are considered as confident samples of the model as defined by the projected features from the training dataset. Unseen data is projected onto a standard feature space and passed through the outlier detector. The unseen data is not touched during training and only given to the model for model prediction. The model is considered to be confident on predictions on inlier samples as those samples are expected to be similar to the training dataset. Otherwise, the model is not expected to be confident, and we cannot rely on the model's prediction. To evaluate the proposed approach, several datasets are used in this paper: the Modified National Institute of Standards and Technology (MNIST) handwritten digits [11] as training data with the United States Postal Service (USPS) [12] and Street View House Number (SVHN) [13] digit datasets as test data, and the National Institutes of Health (NIH) Chest X-ray dataset [14] as training data with private test datasets across three U.S. and Canada hospitals. Three state-of-art DNN networks including VGG16 [10], ResNet50 [15] and DenseNet121 [16] were employed to evaluate the generalizability of this approach.

2 Methods

For an unseen dataset, a DNN model is expected to maintain consistent performance on data that are similar or close to training data. In order to compare training data to unseen data, it is beneficial to project those datasets onto a standard feature space as shown in the literature [7]. In this study, we utilize the ImageNet feature space as our standard feature space. A model is expected to have consistent performance on data that are close to the training data in the ImageNet feature space. The workflow of proposed method is shown in Fig. 2. When a new unseen sample is given, first, it is projected onto the ImageNet feature space to generate a feature vector. Second, the outlier detector predicts whether the unseen data sample is an inlier (close to training dataset) or an outlier (far from training dataset). It is noted that a data-driven model learns common patterns from most samples within a group or class and that outlier samples are more often associated with wrong predictions. We expect a DNN model to maintain consistent performance on inliers when compared to the performance on test samples from the same distribution as the training data.

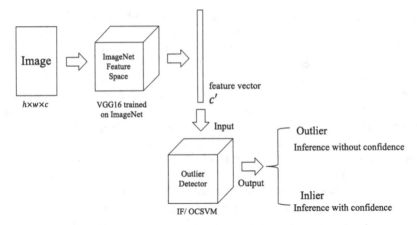

Fig. 2. Illustration of the proposed method.

2.1 Standard Feature Space

To evaluate the similarity between two image datasets, Salimans et al. [7] first proposed the Inception Score (IS), which is computed by projecting both image datasets onto the ImageNet label space using an ImageNet pre-trained Inception model [17]. Images are projected onto this standard space because ImageNet provides 1000 categories of classification labels and it has been shown that it is more reliable to calculate entropies over classification labels in a standard space. Later, Heusel et al. [8] proposed the Fréchet Inception Distance (FID) to improve the consistency of the IS. They used the features from coding layers instead of classification labels to obtain vision-relevant features. The Fréchet distance is calculated from this standard feature space to improve the consistency of similarity measurements across two image datasets.

Borrowing the same idea, to better measure the similarity between the training data and the unseen data, we project our images onto the ImageNet feature space. Due to the page limit, only the results of the standard feature space built on the VGG16 network pretrained on ImageNet are shown in this paper. Results using the ResNet50, Dense-Net121 and InceptionV3 pre-trained ImageNet standard feature spaces are given in the Supplementary Material.

2.2 Outlier Detector

Both IS and FID explicitly measure the distribution similarity between two image sets. However, a large number of images, on the order of thousands of samples, is required to accurately estimate the similarity measurement. In this paper, we aim to identify the similarity of each individual case from an unseen data source against the training dataset. As such, IS and FID cannot be applied here. Therefore, we employ an outlier detection method to classify the data into inliers and outliers to inexplicitly measure the distance between individual cases from an unseen data source and the training dataset.

State of art outlier detector methods in the literature include Isolation Forest (IF) [18] and one-class support vector machine (OCSVM) [19]. IF algorithm is a powerful unsupervised ensemble method for outlier detection based on decision trees. The averaged random tree path length determines whether a data point is an inlier or an outlier. OCSVM identifies the smallest hypersphere consisting of all the data. Data points that fall inside the hypersphere are considered to be inliers, whereas data points outside the hypersphere are considered to be outliers.

In this study, we employed and compared both IF and OCSVM to detect inliers and outliers from unseen data against the training dataset. To construct the outlier detector, only correctly predicted training samples using DNN models are projected onto a standard feature space (ImageNet feature space). The outlier detector is built on these extracted features and is given an outlier ratio, which is defined as the proportion of outliers present in the training data. The outlier ratio helps the outlier detector define the decision boundary to determine outlier data points.

Samples classified as inliers by the outlier detector are considered as confident samples for the DNN models. For the unseen data, model performance is evaluated on the confident samples to evaluate performance improvement on such samples. Detailed experiments will be discussed in next section.

3 Experiments

To validate the proposed method, two sets of experiments were conducted on the MNIST classification [11] and NIH chest X-ray lung field classification tasks [20]. To address these classification tasks, state of the art DNN models including VGG16, ResNet50 and DenseNet121 networks were retrained on the training datasets. The ResNet50, DenseNet121 and VGG16 models were initialized with pre-trained ImageNet weights. In each case, the training process followed the standard training process in Keras [21] with both horizontal and vertical random flipping augmentation during training. The Adam optimizer [22] with a default learning rate of 0.001 was used during training. After the DNN models were trained and tested, the correctly predicted images from the training dataset were projected into the standard space to extract features as stated in Sect. 2. IF and OCSVM outlier detector models were constructed with those extracted features and used to remove outliers. Outlier ratios of 0.1, 0.2, 0.3, 0.4 and 0.5 were selected. Other settings of IF and OCSVM were based on default settings from the Python Scikit-Learn package.

3.1 MNIST Classification

MNIST classification is a classical machine learning task that classifies handwritten digit images into 10 classes (numbers 0 to 9). First, we built MNIST classification models based on VGG16, ResNet50 and DenseNet121. Second, we evaluated those models separately on the MNIST test, USPS and SVHN datasets. As shown in Fig. 3, the USPS dataset [12] is more visually similar to the MNIST dataset while the SVHN dataset [13] is very different. The results reported in Table 1 indicate that the models trained on MNSIT dataset performed reasonably well on USPS data but performed poorly on SVHN dataset.

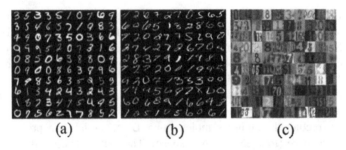

Fig. 3. Sample images from (a) MNIST, (b) USPS, and (c) SVHN datasets.

Benchmark Experimental Results. We benchmark the performance of the DNN models on unseen data. Benchmark accuracy is defined as the classification accuracy of the retrained DNN model on the entire unseen dataset before outlier detection. From Table 1, we observe that the model performance dropped substantially on the unseen USPS and SVHN datasets when compared to the MNIST test dataset. For the ResNet50 model, the accuracy dropped by 16.23% and 77.94% from the MNIST test dataset to the USPS and SVHN datasets, respectively. For DenseNet121, the accuracy dropped by 8.18% and 80.79% from MNIST test dataset to the USPS and SVHN datasets, respectively. For VGG16, the accuracy dropped by 6.54% and 65.97% from MNIST test dataset to the USPS and SVHN datasets, respectively. This reduction in model performance indicates a failure to generalize to unseen data.

Table 1. Performance of the proposed method on the MNIST test, USPS and SVHN datasets

MNIST test data		ResNet50 (99.53%)					DenseNet121 (99.67%)					VGG16 (99.66%)				
Outlier ratio		0.1	0.2	0.3	0.4	0.5	0.1	0.2	0.3	0.4	0.5	0.1	0.2	0.3	0.4	0.5
IF	In	99.54	99.57	99.61	99.59	99.69	99.68	99.72	99.68	99.66	99.73	99.67	99.68	99.66	99.69	99.72
	Out	99.47	99.36	99.33	99.43	99.36	99.53	99.48	99.65	99.69	99.61	99.57	99.59	99.66	99.62	99.59
OCSVM	In	99.53	99.57	99.55	99.62	99.61	99.69	99.68	99.66	99.69	99.69	99.66	99.66	99.66	99.68	99.66
	Out	99.49	99.38	99.48	99.39	99.45	99.49	99.64	99.69	99.64	99.65	99.7	99.65	99.66	99.63	99.66
USPS benchmark		ResNet50 (83.30%)					DenseNet121 (91.49%)					VGG16 (93.12%)				
Outlier ratio		0.1	0.2	0.3	0.4	0.5	0.1	0.2	0.3	0.4	0.5	0.1	0.2	0.3	0.4	0.5
IF	In	83.53	83.82	84.34	85.09	85.87	91.61	91.65	91.77	91.93	92.34	93.07	93.06	93.12	93.28	93.63
	Out	81.88	81.6	81.14	80.87	80.91	90.64	90.92	90.85	90.84	90.62	93.4	93.29	93.11	92.91	92.66
OCSVM	In	83.61	83.63	84.41	85.25	86.59	91.37	91.09	90.9	90.93	91.54	92.98	92.81	92.71	92.9	93.54
	Out	81.87	82.55	81.63	81.4	81.26	92.04	92.44	92.36	92.03	91.46	93.8	93.86	93.74	93.33	92.86
SVHN benchmark		ResNet50 (21.59%)					DenseNet121 (18.88%)					VGG16 (33.69%)				
Outlier ratio		0.1	0.2	0.3	0.4	0.5	0.1	0.2	0.3	0.4	0.5	0.1	0.2	0.3	0.4	0.5
IF	In	50	100	–	–	–	33.33	100	–	–	–	60	–	–	–	–
	Out	21.56	21.58	21.59	21.59	21.59	18.87	18.87	18.88	18.88	18.88	33.68	33.69	33.69	33.69	33.69
OCSVM	In	83.33	100	100	–	–	75	66.67	100	–	–	100	100	100	–	–
	Out	21.55	21.57	21.58	21.59	21.59	18.86	18.87	18.87	18.88	18.88	33.65	33.68	33.68	33.69	33.69

Experimental Results on Inliers. When applying the proposed method, results in Table 1 show that model performance generally improved on confident samples (inliers) when using both IF and OCSVM outlier detectors across different outlier ratios. For the IF outlier detector when compared to benchmark, ResNet50 accuracy improved from 83.30% up to 85.87% on USPS data and 21.59% up to 100% on SVHN data. Similarly, for the OCSVM detector, ResNet50 accuracy improved from 83.30% up to 86.59% on USPS data and 21.59% up to 100% on SVHN data. Similar trends were observed for DenseNet121 and VGG16 (Table 1). The above results empirically support our hypothesis that a generic model will perform consistently well on inlier data. The number of inliers and outliers detected for each dataset are given in the Supplementary Material (Tables S4–S6).

3.2   Chest X-ray Lung Field Classification

The chest frontal X-ray lung field classification was chosen to evaluate the performance of the proposed method. Determination of the acceptability of a patient positioning is one of the key components for successful Quality Control (QC) in a radiology department workflow. All clipped chest X-ray lung field images were considered to belong to the bad lung field class. Figure 1 shows examples of good and bad lung field chest X-ray images from different data sources.

As in the MNIST experiment, the ResNet50, DenseNet121 and VGG16 were selected and trained on the NIH chest X-ray dataset. Three additional datasets from different hospitals across the U.S. and Canada were collected as unseen datasets to evaluate the proposed method. Due to the data contracts, the names of those three hospitals were anonymized to Source 1, Source 2 and Source 3 in this paper.

The NIH dataset had over 112,000 of images from more than 30,000 patients, including many with advanced lung diseases. We selected and manually annotated 7,856 images with good lung field where the whole lung field was clearly visible without any clipping. Manual annotation was performed with the help of Radiology Technologists. In the same manner, 4,356 images with bad lung field were also selected. All the models were trained only on the NIH X-ray dataset with a random split of 75%/15%/15% for training/validation/testing. The three other datasets from Sources 1, 2 and 3 were selected and manually annotated with the same criteria and used as unseen datasets.

Benchmark Experimental Results. From Fig. 4, we observe that the model benchmark accuracy dropped substantially on the unseen datasets from Source 1, 2 and 3 when compared to the NIH test dataset benchmark accuracy. For the ResNet50 model, the accuracy performance dropped by 8.19%, 20.09% and 7.86% from the NIH test dataset on Sources 1, 2 and 3, respectively. For DenseNet121, the accuracy performance dropped by 8.31%, 19.64% and 6.03% from the NIH test dataset on Sources 1, 2 and 3, respectively. For VGG16, the accuracy performance dropped by 7.80%, 14.13% and 7.02% from the NIH test dataset on Sources 1, 2 and 3, respectively.

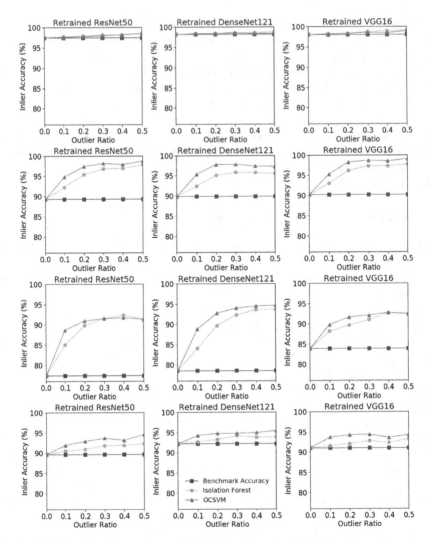

Fig. 4. Inlier classification accuracy (%) as a function of outlier ratio across X-ray image datasets originating from (a) NIH test, (b) Source 1, (c) Source 2 and (d) Source 3. Benchmark accuracy is defined as the classification accuracy of the retrained DNN model on the entire unseen dataset before outlier detection.

Experimental Results on Inliers. While applying the proposed method, results in Fig. 4 show that the performance of all models improved for both IF and OCSVM across different outlier ratios. When using IF as the outlier detector, the ResNet50 accuracy improved from 89.30%, 77.40% and 89.63% up to 97.75%, 92.35% and 92.29% on Sources 1, 2 and 3, respectively. DenseNet121 accuracy improved from 89.89%, 78.56% and 92.17% up to 95.75%, 93.64% and 94.21% on Sources 1, 2 and 3, respectively. VGG16 accuracy improved from 90.23%, 83.90% and 91.01% up to

97.75%, 92.71% and 93.31% on Sources 1, 2 and 3 respectively. By using OCSVM, the best accuracy that ResNet50 can achieve is up to 98.77%, 91.73% and 94.61% on Sources 1, 2 and 3, respectively. The best accuracy that DenseNet121 can achieve is up to 97.78%, 94.66% and 95.42% on Sources 1, 2 and 3, respectively. The best accuracy that VGG16 can achieve is 99.08%, 92.73% and 94.45% on data Sources 1, 2 and 3, respectively. Similar to the experimental results on the MNIST digit images, the experimental results on medical chest X-ray images also show that a generic model performed better on its confident samples (inliers) across different outlier detectors. The number of inliers and outliers detected for each dataset are given in the Supplementary Material (Tables S11–S14).

4   Discussion and Conclusion

As observed in both Table 1 and Fig. 4, the model has improved performance on the inliers of unseen data despite the fact that the model would typically not be confident on most of the samples in the unseen datasets. This can help clinicians prioritize and allocate more resources to cases where the model is not confident. However, the quality of proposed method heavily depends on the robustness of feature extractors and the outlier detectors that are used. In this paper, we consider the feature space constructed from the VGG16 network trained on ImageNet. Additionally, based on our preliminary experiments, we have noticed that when the outlier detector was not well constructed, the inliers identified were not implying correct predictions. One potential way to resolve these issues, which is one of our future work is to build an end-to-end framework incorporating both Bayesian approach (resolves uncertainty) and outlier detection (resolves domain-shift).

In this study, we proposed a novel method to determine the confident samples. An outlier detection model was constructed based on the features extracted from the standard feature space. Inliers from the detection model were considered as the confident samples from the unseen data. Experimental results showed that the performance of the ResNet50, DenseNet121 and VGG16 models improved on all unseen datasets after filtering out outliers.

References

1. Chen, T., Navrátil, J., Iyengar, V., Shanmugam, K.: Confidence scoring using whitebox meta-models with linear classifier probes. arXiv preprint arXiv:1805.05396 (2018)
2. Gal, Y., Ghahramani, Z.: Dropout as a bayesian approximation: representing model uncertainty in deep learning. In: International Conference on Machine Learning, pp. 1050–1059 (2016)
3. Nair, T., Precup, D., Arnold, D.L., Arbel, T.: Exploring uncertainty measures in deep networks for multiple sclerosis lesion detection and segmentation. In: Frangi, A.F., Schnabel, J.A., Davatzikos, C., Alberola-López, C., Fichtinger, G. (eds.) MICCAI 2018. LNCS, vol. 11070, pp. 655–663. Springer, Cham (2018). https://doi.org/10.1007/978-3-030-00928-1_74

4. Leibig, C., Allken, V., Ayhan, M.S., Berens, P., Wahl, S.: Leveraging uncertainty information from deep neural networks for disease detection. Sci. Rep. **7**, 17816 (2017)
5. Geifman, Y., El-Yaniv, R.: Selective classification for deep neural networks. In: Advances in Neural Information Processing Systems, pp. 4878–4887 (2017)
6. Hendrycks, D., Gimpel, K.: A baseline for detecting misclassified and out-of-distribution examples in neural networks. arXiv preprint arXiv:1610.02136 (2016)
7. Salimans, T., Goodfellow, I., Zaremba, W., Cheung, V., Radford, A., Chen, X.: Improved techniques for training GANs. In: Advances in Neural Information Processing Systems, pp. 2234–2242 (2016)
8. Heusel, M., Ramsauer, H., Unterthiner, T., Nessler, B., Hochreiter, S.: GANs trained by a two time-scale update rule converge to a local Nash equilibrium. In: Advances in Neural Information Processing Systems, pp. 6626–6637 (2017)
9. Deng, J., Dong, W., Socher, R., Li, L.-J., Li, K., Fei-Fei, L.: ImageNet: a large-scale hierarchical image database. In: 2009 IEEE Conference on Computer Vision and Pattern Recognition, pp. 248–255. IEEE (2009)
10. Simonyan, K., Zisserman, A.: Very deep convolutional networks for large-scale image recognition. arXiv preprint arXiv:1409.1556 (2014)
11. LeCun, Y., Bottou, L., Bengio, Y., Haffner, P.: Gradient-based learning applied to document recognition. Proc. IEEE **86**, 2278–2324 (1998)
12. Hull, J.J.: A database for handwritten text recognition research. IEEE Trans. Pattern Anal. Mach. Intell. **16**, 550–554 (1994)
13. Netzer, Y., Wang, T., Coates, A., Bissacco, A., Wu, B., Ng, A.Y.: Reading digits in natural images with unsupervised feature learning (2011)
14. Wang, X., Peng, Y., Lu, L., Lu, Z., Bagheri, M., Summers, R.M.: Chestx-ray8: hospital-scale chest x-ray database and benchmarks on weakly-supervised classification and localization of common thorax diseases. In: Proceedings of the IEEE Conference on Computer Vision and Pattern Recognition, pp. 2097–2106 (2017)
15. He, K., Zhang, X., Ren, S., Sun, J.: Deep residual learning for image recognition. In: Proceedings of the IEEE Conference on Computer Vision and Pattern Recognition, pp. 770–778 (2016)
16. Huang, G., Liu, Z., Van Der Maaten, L., Weinberger, K.Q.: Densely connected convolutional networks. In: Proceedings of the IEEE Conference on Computer Vision and Pattern Recognition, pp. 4700–4708 (2017)
17. Szegedy, C., Vanhoucke, V., Ioffe, S., Shlens, J., Wojna, Z.: Rethinking the inception architecture for computer vision. In: Proceedings of the IEEE Conference on Computer Vision and Pattern Recognition, pp. 2818–2826 (2016)
18. Liu, F.T., Ting, K.M., Zhou, Z.-H.: Isolation forest. In: 2008 Eighth IEEE International Conference on Data Mining, pp. 413–422. IEEE (2008)
19. Moya, M.M., Hush, D.R.: Network constraints and multi-objective optimization for one-class classification. Neural Networks. **9**, 463–474 (1996)
20. Competition, B.P.: AAPM spring clinical meeting-abstracts SATURDAY, APRIL 7. J. Appl. Clin. Med. Phys. **19**, 370–407 (2018)
21. Chollet, F.: Deep Learning mit Python und Keras: Das Praxis-Handbuch vom Entwickler der Keras-Bibliothek. MITP-Verlags GmbH & Co. KG (2018)
22. Kingma, D.P., Ba, J.: Adam: a method for stochastic optimization. arXiv preprint arXiv: 1412.6980 (2014)

Out of Distribution Detection for Intra-operative Functional Imaging

Tim J. Adler[1,2]([envelope]), Leonardo Ayala[1], Lynton Ardizzone[3],
Hannes G. Kenngott[4], Anant Vemuri[1], Beat P. Müller-Stich[4], Carsten Rother[3],
Ullrich Köthe[3], and Lena Maier-Hein[1]([envelope])

[1] Division Computer Assisted Medical Interventions (CAMI), German Cancer
Research Center (DKFZ), Heidelberg, Germany
{t.adler,l.maier-hein}@dkfz.de
[2] Faculty of Mathematics and Computer Science, Heidelberg University,
Heidelberg, Germany
[3] Visual Learning Lab, Heidelberg University, Heidelberg, Germany
[4] Division of Minimally-invasive Surgery of the Department of General Surgery,
Heidelberg University, Heidelberg, Germany

Abstract. Multispectral optical imaging is becoming a key tool in the
operating room. Recent research has shown that machine learning algorithms can be used to convert pixel-wise reflectance measurements to
tissue parameters, such as oxygenation. However, the accuracy of these
algorithms can only be guaranteed if the spectra acquired during surgery
match the ones seen during training. It is therefore of great interest to
detect so-called *out of distribution* (OoD) spectra to prevent the algorithm from presenting spurious results. In this paper we present an information theory based approach to OoD detection based on the *widely
applicable information criterion* (WAIC). Our work builds upon recent
methodology related to *invertible neural networks* (INN). Specifically, we
make use of an ensemble of INNs as we need their tractable Jacobians in
order to compute the WAIC. Comprehensive experiments with *in silico*,
and *in vivo* multispectral imaging data indicate that our approach is
well-suited for OoD detection. Our method could thus be an important
step towards reliable functional imaging in the operating room.

1 Introduction

The most commonly applied approach to computer aided surgery (CAS) relies
on fusing pre-operative medical images with the current patient anatomy for
augmented reality guidance. While this approach is well-suited for displaying
subsurface structures detected in pre-operative images, such as tumors or vessels,
a main bottleneck is the fact that it cannot account for tissue dynamics; live
monitoring of perfusion, for example, is not possible with an approach that relies
on 'offline images'. To address this shortcoming, recent research has focused on
intra-operative functional imaging using biophotonics techniques. In this context,
multispectral optical imaging is evolving as a key tool. Previous work has shown

© Springer Nature Switzerland AG 2019
H. Greenspan et al. (Eds.): CLIP 2019/UNSURE 2019, LNCS 11840, pp. 75–82, 2019.
https://doi.org/10.1007/978-3-030-32689-0_8

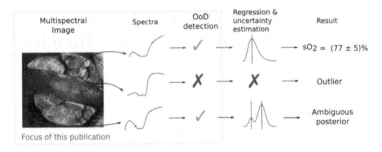

Fig. 1. Proposed multi-stage process for uncertainty handling in multispectral image analysis. To investigate whether the input (here: a spectrum) is sufficiently close to the training data, *out of distribution* (OoD) detection is performed. If the input is regarded as valid, the corresponding functional tissue parameters are computed. To address the potential inherent ambiguity of the problem a full posterior probability distribution rather than a point estimate is provided for each tissue parameter (here: blood oxygenation).

that machine learning algorithms can be used to convert pixel-wise reflectance measurements to tissue parameters, such as oxygenation [13,14]. These methods learn to infer tissue parameters via training samples providing a spectrum and the correct corresponding tissue parameter(s) (supervised learning). However, the accuracy of these algorithms is heavily effected by aleatoric and epistemic uncertainties [6].

In this paper, we argue for a multi-stage process for uncertainty handling as illustrated in Fig. 1. (1) To investigate whether the input is sufficiently close to the training data, *out of distribution* (OoD) detection is performed. (2) If the input is regarded as valid, the corresponding functional tissue parameters are computed, and a full posterior probability distribution is provided as output for each tissue parameter. As the second part of this pipeline has already been addressed in recent publications [1,2], we will focus on the first part. The following sections present and validate our proposed approach to OoD detection.

2   Methods

While we are not aware of any previous work in OoD detection in the field of optical imaging, the topic has gained increasing interest in the machine learning community. To implement the proposed multi-stage process for uncertainty handling in multispectral image analysis (Fig. 1), we build our method upon the work by Choi et al. [3] who proposed the *widely applicable information criterion* (WAIC) as a means to measure the closeness of a new sample to the training distribution. The advantage of this method lies in the fact that it outperforms many other ensemble based unsupervised learning methods while still being easily computable. An unsupervised approach is integral to the method as it is not feasible to generate enough labeled negative samples to train a discriminator between in- and outliers [3,10]. The challenge in applying WAIC is the fact that it is an ensemble based method leading to the necessity of training a model multiple times. Depending on the data dimensions this can become prohibitively expensive both in terms of time and hardware requirements. In this work, we use invertible neural networks (INN) [2] to estimate WAIC on multispectral endoscopic imaging data.

In this section, we briefly revisit WAIC [3] and give an intuition for this quantity (Sect. 2.1), present the INN architecture as an integral ingredient to apply WAIC in the surgical domain (Sect. 2.2) and describe our experimental validation (Sect. 2.3).

2.1   Principle of WAIC

In the original contribution [12], WAIC is defined as

$$\text{WAIC}(x) = \text{Var}_\Theta[\log p(x \mid \Theta)] - \mathbb{E}_\Theta[\log p(x \mid \Theta)], \tag{1}$$

where $\text{WAIC}(x)$ quantifies the proximity of a sample x to the distribution of the training data X^{tr}, and Θ is distributed according to $p(\Theta \mid X^{\text{tr}})$. In a very recent publication [3] it was suggested to use WAIC as a means for OoD in the setting of neural networks.[1] The variance term in Eq. (1) measures 'how certain' the posterior distribution $p(\cdot \mid \Theta)$ is about a sample x, the heuristic being that it should be more certain about samples that are close to what it has seen before. The expectation term in Eq. (1) is used for normalization. The idea is that if the expectation of $\log p(x \mid \Theta)$ is high then the spread measured by the variance might also be larger without really measuring internal uncertainty of the model. Hence, it is subtracted to account for this effect.

2.2   WAIC Computation with INNs

WAIC only works for parametrized models. To meet this precondition, we use a deep neural network to encode the spectra X in a latent space Z following an analytically tractable distribution, which we chose to be a multivariate standard Gaussian. Let $f_\Theta : X \subset \mathbb{R}^n \to Z \subset \mathbb{R}^n$ denote the the neural network with parameters Θ. Then we can use the change of variable formula to compute the log-likelihood $\log p(x \mid \Theta)$ for a spectrum x as

$$\log p(x \mid \Theta) = -\frac{1}{2}\|f_\Theta(x)\|_2^2 - \frac{n}{2}\log(2\pi) + \log|\det Jf_\Theta(x)|, \tag{2}$$

where Jf_Θ denotes its Jacobian [11]. Equation (2) shows that it is mandatory for the log-Jacobi determinant of our network to be efficiently computable. One established architecture is the one of *normalizing flows* originally introduced in [4] and refined in [2] under the name of *invertible neural networks* (INN). For

---

[1] Please note that the sign convention of WAIC of Choi and Watanabe are opposite. We chose Watanabe's definition.

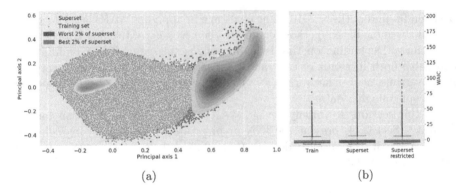

(a)   (b)

Fig. 2. In silico validation. (a) The WAIC method trained on the training set (turquoise points, here projected onto the first two principal components (PCA) of the complete training set X_{SC}^{tr}) was applied to the superset (here: blue points). The 2% percentile of best and worst superset spectra according the WAIC value are shown as a kernel density estimation in green (representing *in distribution* samples) and red (representing *out of distribution* samples) respectively. (b) The WAIC distribution of the training set, superset and restricted superset is shown (superset boxplot truncated).

each of the experiments described in the next section, we trained an ensemble of INNs to estimate $p(\Theta \mid X^{tr})$. Each network consisted of 10 layers of so called coupling blocks (see [4]) each followed by a permutation layer. Each coupling block consisted of a 3 layer fully connected network with ReLU activation functions. The networks were trained using Maximum-Likelihood training, i.e. by minimizing the loss $L(x) = -\log p(x \mid \Theta)$ as given in Eq. (2) using the Adam optimizer [7].

2.3   Experiments

The purpose of our experiments was to validate our approach to OoD detection *in silico* (Sect. 2.3), and to present *in vivo* use cases (Sect. 2.3).

In Silico Quantitative Validation. In our simulation framework, a multi-spectral imaging pixel is generated from a 8-valued vector $\mathbf{t}_i$ of tissue properties, which are assumed to be relevant for the image formation process. Plausible tissue samples $\mathbf{t}_i$, are drawn from a layered tissue model as proposed in [14]. The framework was used to generate a data set X_{raw}, consisting of 550,000 high resolution spectra and corresponding ground truth tissue properties. It was split in a training X_{raw}^{tr} and test set X_{raw}^{te}, comprising 500,000 and 50,000 spectra respectively. For the *in silico* quantitative validation we converted the (high resolution) spectra of the simulated data sets to plausible camera measurements using the filter response functions of the 8-band Pixelteq SpectroCam. We use a subscript (here: SC for SpectroCam) to refer to the data set X_{raw} after it was adapted to a certain camera. X_{SC}^{tr} was split into a small training set $X_{SC}^{tr,s}$ and a *superset* $X_{\text{SC}}^{\text{sup}}$, such that the support of $X_{\text{SC}}^{\text{tr,s}}$ lay within the support of $X_{\text{SC}}^{\text{sup}}$ and $X_{\text{SC}}^{\text{sup}}$ consisted of a cluster of data points outside of the support of $X_{\text{SC}}^{\text{tr,s}}$, as illustrated in Fig. 2 (a). This led to a split of $X_{\text{SC}}^{\text{tr,d}}$ of approximately 49% of $X_{\text{SC}}^{\text{tr}}$ and $X_{\text{SC}}^{\text{sup}}$ of approximately 51% of $X_{\text{SC}}^{\text{tr}}$. An ensemble of five INNs was trained on $X_{\text{SC}}^{\text{tr,s}}$ and the WAIC value was evaluated on $X_{\text{SC}}^{\text{sup}}$. We defined $X_{\text{SC}}^{\text{sup,r}}$ as the *reduced* data set of $X_{\text{SC}}^{\text{sup}}$ lying in the support of $X_{\text{SC}}^{\text{tr,s}}$. We then investigated (1) whether the WAIC distribution of the $X_{\text{SC}}^{\text{sup,r}}$ matches that of the $X_{\text{SC}}^{\text{tr,s}}$ and whether (2) the part of $X_{\text{SC}}^{\text{sup}}$ not in the support of $X_{\text{SC}}^{\text{tr,s}}$ was correctly classified as outliers by our method.

In Vivo Application. While the goal of the previous experiment was to confirm the validity of our approach in an *in silico* setting, the purpose of the *in vivo* experiments were to showcase applications in which the OoD detection could be useful.

Anomaly/Novelty Detection: Detecting (parts of) a multispectral image in which the spectra do not closely match the training data distribution can be useful for many reasons. Possible applications include the detection of abnormal tissue or of artifical objects (e. g. instruments). To investigate this aspect, we used the complete $X_{\text{SC}}^{\text{tr}}$ to train an ensemble of five INNs. As *in vivo* test data, we acquired endoscopic images of porcine organs which we classified as *organs lying in the simulation domain* X^{iD} and *organs not lying in the simulation domain* X^{oD}. These spectra were acquired using a Pixelteq SpectroCam on a 30° Stortz laparascope with a Stortz Xenon light source (Storz D-light P 201337 20). We classified liver, spleen, abdominal wall, diaphragm and bowl as in domain organs as hemoglobin can be assumed to be the main absorber in these. In contrast, we classified gallbladder as an out of domain organ, since bile is a notable absorber but has not been considered in our simulation framework. With this, X^{iD} and X^{oD} consisted of 50000 spectra and 10000 spectra respectively. Our hypothesis was that the WAIC values of X^{iD} should be much lower than those for X^{oD}. For reference, we also compared the resulting WAIC distributions to that of the simulated test data $X_{\text{SC}}^{\text{te}}$.

Detection of Scene Changes: Intra-operative image modalities often rely on a careful calibration of the device. When recovering blood oxygenation from multispectral measurements, for example, the regressor is typically trained with the light source that is used during test time. To investigate whether WAIC is applicable to detect illumination changes (which would substantially harm the method and render the estimation results invalid), we adapted X_{raw} to a xiQ XIMEA (Muenster, Germany) $SNm4 \times 4$ mosaic camera consisting of 16 bands assuming a Wolf LED light source (Wolf Endolight LED 2.2). We trained an ensemble of five INNs on $X_{\text{Xim}}^{\text{tr}}$. Furthermore, we recorded 200 512×272-pixel images of the lip of a healthy human volunteer using the xiQ XIMEA camera and a 30° Stortz laparascope (cf. Fig. 4(b)). At around image 80 we switched the endoscope from a Stortz Xenon light source (Storz D-light P 201337 20) to a Wolf LED light source (Wolf Endolight LED 2.2). Based on the hypothesis that the switch in light source would be detected by WAIC analysis, we computed the WAIC time series for the region of interest depicted in Fig. 4(a).

3   Results

In Silico Validation. The distribution of the reduced training data $X_{SC}^{tr,s}$ and the superset X_{SC}^{sup} (projected to the first two principal components) can be found in Fig. 2(a). It can be seen that the samples with poor WAIC values (red) concentrate in the superset part not contained in $X_{SC}^{tr,s}$, whereas samples with low WAIC values (green) are contained in the interior of $X_{SC}^{tr,s}$. Figure 2(b) shows a comparison between the WAIC distributions of $X_{SC}^{tr,s}$, X_{SC}^{sup} and the restricted superset $X_{SC}^{sup,r}$. The data sets $X_{SC}^{tr,s}$ and $X_{SC}^{sup,r}$ are in excellent agreement. The superset X_{SC}^{sup} only differs in the regard that there are far more outliers, which can be accounted to the data points outside of $X_{SC}^{tr,s}$.

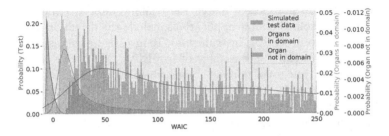

Fig. 3. Histogram of the WAIC values for the simulated test set, and *in vivo* multispectral measurements of organs that do (green) or do not (red) match the model assumptions based on which the training data was generated (tails truncated). Please note the different scales for the three distributions. (Color figure online)

Application. The WAIC distribution for the test data X_{SC}^{te}, the *in domain organs* X^{iD} and the *out of domain organ* X^{oD} can be found in Fig. 3. The distribution of the test data is by far the sharpest with a maximum a posterior probability (MAP) at -4.9. The distribution closely matches that of the training data (MAP $= -4.9$). The distribution of X^{iD} also possesses a sharp maximum, however with a far heavier tail. The MAP estimate yields 9.3 which indicates a still existent domain gap between our simulation domain and the organ domain. The distribution of X^{oD} is very noisy and has an even heavier tail than X^{iD}. The MAP lies at 34. This indicates that our WAIC estimate is suitable to distinguish between in domain tissue and out of domain tissue. Similarly, Fig. 4 illustrates that the change in illumination as performed in the *detection of scence changes* experiment results in a drastic change of WAIC values.

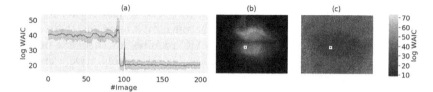

Fig. 4. Automatic detection of scene changes. (a) When a change in light source occurs, the mean log WAIC values computed for the white region of interest in (b)/(c) drop, indicating a decreasing domain gap between training and test data. (b) RGB image estimated using the 8-band measurement of human lips. (c) Corresponding WAIC values computed for the multispectral image. (Color figure online)

4   Discussion

The accuracy of machine learning-based regression methods in multispectral imaging crucially depend on whether the spectra acquired during surgery match the ones seen during training. Although initial steps with respect to uncertainty estimation and compensation have been taken in the field of optical imaging [1, 2,5,8,9,15], we are, to our knowledge, the first to address the problem of OoD detection to prevent algorithms from presenting spurious results.

The application to endoscopic organ data showed that our method is well-suited for anomaly detection. The in distribution organs are well separated from the out of distribution organ (gallbladder). Moreover, this experiment reveals a shortcoming of the simulation framework proposed by [14]: The large difference in the WAIC distribution between the test set and the real data indicates a domain gap that remains to be tackled.

Our experiments with human lips show that WAIC is able to distinguish between different lighting conditions. The uncertainty prior to the change of lighting can most likely be explained by the short darkness stemming from the light source switch. The jump at image 100 was due to involuntary movement of the volunteer leading to the image being out of focus. One reason for the generally high WAIC values is the fact that melanin (a chromophore in the skin) was not simulated in the training data.

In the present implementation we used five INNs in our ensembles. According to preliminary experiments, this number is sufficient. We computed the WAIC on the data sets used for the anomality detection experiment (Sect. 2.3) for up to 20 ensemble members. For both the simulated test data and the in domain organs the values stabilized below $n = 10$. For the out of domain data (gallbladder) the WAIC values increased throughout. This merits further investigation. However, there should be no impact on the method performance, as X^{iD} and X^{oD} were well separated.

Our findings underline the power of WAIC in the setting of medical OoD detection. However, there are still some open questions. A general downside of WAIC is its 'arbitrary units' and it is not straightforward to define a threshold for outlier detection. One approach to tackle this shortcoming would be to find a suitable normalization. Another possibility might be to just mask the worst n pixels in a certain ROI. Additionally, to this conceptual question, there are also practical limitations. The estimation of WAIC requires an *ensemble* of neural networks, which was feasible in our case, but becomes prohibitively expensive for larger input dimensions. For the future, methods for network compression might be adapted to tackle this problem.

In conclusion, this paper is the first to address the topic of OoD detection in intra-operative imaging. Due to the promising results obtained in this study, the approach proposed could not only become a valuable tool for increasing the reliability of machine learning-based regression methods but could also boost research in unsupervised intra-operative anomaly detection.

References

1. Adler, T.J., et al.: Uncertainty-aware performance assessment of optical imaging modalities with invertible neural networks. Int. J. Comput. Assist. Radiol. Surg. (2019)
2. Ardizzone, L., Kruse, J., Rother, C., Köthe, U.: Analyzing inverse problems with invertible neural networks. In: International Conference on Learning Representations (2019)
3. Choi, H., Jang, E., Alemi, A.A.: Waic, but why? Generative ensembles for robust anomaly detection. CoRR (2018)
4. Dinh, L., Sohl-Dickstein, J., Bengio, S.: Density estimation using Real NVP. CoRR (2016)
5. Gal, Y., Ghahramani, Z.: Dropout as a Bayesian approximation: representing Model Uncertainty in deep learning (2016)
6. Kendall, A., Gal, Y.: What uncertainties do we need in Bayesian deep learning for computer vision? In: Advances in Neural Information Processing Systems, vol. 30. Curran Associates, Inc. (2017)
7. Kingma, D.P., Ba, J.: Adam: A method for stochastic optimization. arXiv preprint arXiv:1412.6980 (2014)
8. Kohl, S.A.A., et al.: A probabilistic U-Net for segmentation of ambiguous images (2018)
9. Leibig, C., Allken, V., Ayhan, M.S., Berens, P., Wahl, S.: Leveraging uncertainty information from deep neural networks for disease detection. Sci. Rep. (2017)
10. Markou, M., Singh, S.: Novelty detection: a reviewpart 1: statistical approaches. Sig. Process. (2003)
11. Walter, R.: Real and Complex Analysis (1987)
12. Watanabe, S.: Algebraic Geometry and Statistical Learning Theory. Cambridge University Press, Cambridge (2009)
13. Wirkert, S.J., et al.: Robust near real-time estimation of physiological parameters from megapixel multispectral images with inverse Monte Carlo and random forest regression. Int. J. Comput. Assist. Radiol. Surg. (2016)
14. Wirkert, S.J., et al.: Physiological parameter estimation from multispectral images unleashed. In: Descoteaux, M., Maier-Hein, L., Franz, A., Jannin, P., Collins, D.L., Duchesne, S. (eds.) MICCAI 2017. LNCS, vol. 10435, pp. 134–141. Springer, Cham (2017). https://doi.org/10.1007/978-3-319-66179-7_16
15. Zhu, Y., Zabaras, N.: Bayesian deep convolutional encoder-decoder networks for surrogate modeling and uncertainty quantification. J. Comput. Phys. (2018)

CLIP 2019

A Clinical Measuring Platform for Building the Bridge Across the Quantification of Pathological N-Cells in Medical Imaging for Studies of Disease

Peifang Guo[(✉)]

Montreal, QC, Canada
peif.guo@gmail.com

Abstract. In this paper, a clinical measuring platform for quantifying nucleus-cells (MPQ-N-cells) at combining a novel color region-based segmentation strategy is proposed to accelerate the discovery of diseases diagnostically in medical imaging. In the approach, average values of colors in an image are employed as similarity criteria to assign image voxels to regions using the minimum distance classifier in the color region growing process. Then, the binary image transformation and graphic contour line procedure are performed, followed by the operation of region area calculation to obtain the actual numbers of voxels within the segmented patterns of the N-cells quantitatively. The proposed approach of MPQ-N-cells is implemented on the heterogeneous medical image datasets related to Parkinson disease, oculopharyngeal muscular dystrophy (one type of protein conformational diseases) and glioblastoma cancer. Implementation results reveal that the proposed MPQ-N-cells approach is capable of quantifying a variety of pathological N-cells clinically with improved data visualization in heterogeneous datasets. This study has the potential to lead to more successful measurement of cell diagnostically and further to track changes of cell in medical imaging for a longitudinal study on supporting the studies of disease.

Keywords: Pathological nucleus cells measurement · Color region-based segmentation · Region area calculation · Binary image transformation · Graphic contour line procedure · Minimum distance classifier · Parkinson disease-related protein · Glioblastoma · Protein conformational diseases

1 Introduction

Numerous human diseases, such as Parkinson disease (PD) and protein conformational diseases (PCDs), have characteristic pathologic signatures involving the accumulation of particular protein as extracellular deposits or intracellular inclusions in certain organs. In general, the deposits of abnormal protein accumulation have the appearance of nucleus-cells (N-cells) in medical imaging (Fereshtehnejad et al. 2017; Tanti et al. 2014; Hortin et al. 2010; Blumen et al. 2009). Medical studies also show that brains of people with glioblastoma cancer, one of the most aggressive malignant primary tumors

© Springer Nature Switzerland AG 2019
H. Greenspan et al. (Eds.): CLIP 2019/UNSURE 2019, LNCS 11840, pp. 85–93, 2019.
https://doi.org/10.1007/978-3-030-32689-0_9

among 120 different types of brain tumors, are composed of spongioblasts with the shape of N-cells pathologically in medical imaging (Raghavendra et al. 2018; Gerard et al. 2017; Egger, et al. 2013; Bauer, et al. 2013).

Medical images in different modality are able to exhibit different characteristic information of human body and pathological changed tissue of N-cells related to diseases. In general, associated with other clinical factors and disease symptoms, the stages of disease could be defined approximately by the degree of N-cells spread in medical imaging. Usually, the higher amounts of pathological N-cells are correlated with aggressive diseases, compared to the early stage cases. Hence, an approach to quantifying pathological N-cells at combing the visualization of segmented N-cells spread in imaging could serve as a stage indicator for a reference in differentiating between early stage and advanced (aggressive) diseases related to PD, PCDs and glioblastoma cancer for disease diagnosis (Guo 2017; Gerard et al., 2017; Blumen et al. 2009).

Due to the presence of image noise in the mage acquisition process, similar characteristics of normal and some abnormal tissue of N-cells may cause interpretational errors in medical imaging. In addition, the huge amount of medical image data produced by imaging devices makes the measurement of potential diseases of N-cells a heavy task in clinical settings (Bakas, et al. 2017; Duyn 2012; Hortin, et al. 2010). It is useful to design a platform for the segmentation of abnormalities of N-cells followed by the measurement of segmented patterns of N-cells subsequently in medical imaging (Guo et al. 2018; Ahmed et al. 2015; Gui et al. 2012). This study seeks to address the issue of measuring pathological N-cells quantitatively at combining a novel color region-based segmentation strategy in the heterogeneous medical imaging, related to PD, one type of PCDs, oculopharyngeal muscular dystrophy (PCDs-OPMD) and glioblastoma cancer on supporting the studies of disease.

2   Proposed Platform

There are different methodologies for image segmentation of N-cells in the literature, including the deep learning based algorithms using image markers (Al-Kofahi et al. 2018; Pärnamaa et al. 2017), the graphical model methods (Murphy 2010; Deshmukh et al. 2014), the threshold-based techniques (Wang et al. 2014; Rafael et al. 2008; Ostu 1979), the level set method (Dzyubachyk et al. 2008). Most of methodologies above rely on the information of shapes of N-cells, which would be applicable only when the appropriate shapes of N-cells in images are available (Rafael et al. 2008; Tohka 2014). Unlike the methodologies of segmentation reviewed above, this study designs the color region-based segmentation strategy to extract disease-related-patterns of N-cells for quantifying segmented patterns of N-cells with irregular shape in medical imaging.

The goal of color region-based segmentation is to divide an image into a set of non-overlapping regions of similar attributes with color. Figure 1 shows a clinical measuring platform for quantifying N-cells (MPQ-N-cells) via a novel strategy of color region-based segmentation with data visualization in medical imaging on supporting the diagnoses of disease. In a color image, each voxel will be represented as a vector of the red, green and blue components (RGB-c) from the origin to that voxel point in the space of RGB-c. Starting from computing the average of colors in the RGB-c for regions of pattern in an image, the proposed MPQ-N-cells then employs the average values of color in the RGB-c as the similarity criterion to assign voxels in regions in the region growing process. When the similarity criterion is satisfied with the minimum distance classifier, the voxel will be assigned in that region, indicating that the voxel most closely matches that color of the region in the space of RGB-c in segmentation.

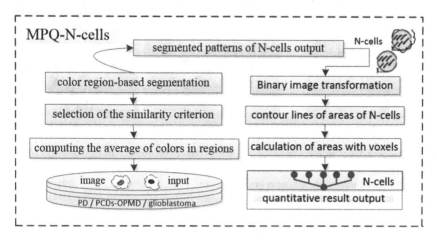

Fig. 1. Proposed platform.

Further, together with the steps of binary image transformation and graphic contour line procedure, the operation of region area calculation is accomplished to obtain the actual numbers of voxels within the segmented patterns of the N-cells quantitatively. In the validation stage, the MPQ-N-cells approach is implemented on heterogeneous medical image datasets, including the PD-related protein image, the microscopy images of PCDs-OPMD and the multi-photon microscopy images of glioblastoma cancer.

3 Implementation Results

The PTEN-induced putative kinase 1 (PINK1) is a serine protein kinase which is implicated in protecting cells from stress-induced mitochondrial dysfunction. Mutations in this gene are thought to be the cause of autosomal recessive early-onset Parkinson disease 6 (PARK6) (Tanti et al. 2014; Hortin et al. 2010). Figure 2 presents the segmentation results from an example of experiments in the MPQ-N-cells implementation in the medical image, where the PD-related protein PINK1 was in the process of presenting mitochondrial antigens with red color for the immune system. Figure 2(a) is the original PD-related protein image (Image credit: The Neuro) with two different colors, red and green. Achieved from the MPQ-N-cells implementation in this study, Fig. 2(b)–(c) are the segmentation results with the output of two extracted image patterns of N-cells, the segmented cell of mitochondrial antigens with red in Fig. 2(b) and the segmented cell of intact mitochondria with green in Fig. 2(c) (both segmented image patterns in Fig. 2(b)–(c) need to be measured quantitatively further in this study).

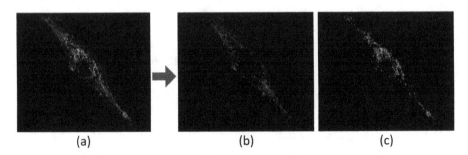

(a)   (b)   (c)

Fig. 2. Segmentation results from an example of experiments from the MPQ-N-cells implementation in the PD-related protein image: (a) original PD-related protein image; (b) segmented mitochondrial antigens with red (c) segmented intact mitochondria with green. (Color figure online) The Neuro

Each proteopathy of PCDs is characterized by a disease-specific buildup of aggregated proteins within tissue of the body. For the type of PCDs, oculopharyngeal muscular dystrophy (PCDs-OPMD), the Poly(A)-Binding Protein 1 (PABPN1) induces the formation of N-cells of muscular intranuclear inclusions (MII) that are the pathological biomarkers of PCDs-OPMD (Blumen et al. 2009; Hortin et al. 2010). Figure 3 shows two examples of the experiments in the MPQ-N-cells implementation on the microscopic image data of PCDs-OPMD. Figure 3(a) is the two original microscopic images of PCDs-OPMD (Image credit: the Centre Hospitalier de l'Université de Montréal), where the N-cells of MII show the light green color. Achieved from the MPQ-N-cells implementation, the segmentation results are shown in Fig. 3(b)–(e) with the output of the four extracted image patterns, the image background with black color in Fig. 3(e), the two layers with various dark green colors in Fig. 3(c)–(d) and the MII cells with light green color in Fig. 3(b) (needs to be measured quantitatively further in this study).

Glioblastoma is a fast-growing malignant brain tumor composed of spongioblasts (Menze et al. 2015; Egger, et al., 2013). Figure 4 shows the segmentation results from two examples of experiments in the MPQ-N-cells implementation in multi-photon microscopy images of glioblastoma. Figure 4(a) is the two original images of glioblastoma (Image credit: Raghavendra et al. 2018) with two different colors of patterns, the glioblastoma cells in green and image markers in white. Achieved from the MPQ-N-cells implementation, the segmentation results are shown in Fig. 4(b)–(c) with the output of the two segmented image patterns, the segmented patterns of markers with white in Fig. 4(c) and the segmented patterns of glioblastoma cells with green in Fig. 4(b) (needs to be measured quantitatively further in this study).

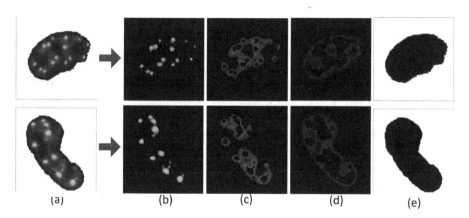

Fig. 3. Segmentation results from two examples of experiments from the MPQ-N-cells implementation on the PCDs-OPMD data: (a) two original microscopic images of PCDs-OPMD; (b) segmented MII cells with light green; (c)–(d) two segmented layers with various dark greens; (e) the background with black. (Color figure online) the Centre Hospitalier de l'Université de Montréal

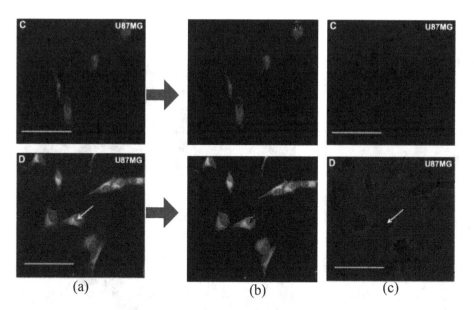

Fig. 4. Segmentation results from two examples of experiments in multi-photon microscopy images of glioblastoma; (a) two original images of glioblastoma; (b)–(c) segmented glioblastoma cells in green and segmented image markers in white, both achieved from the MPQ-N-cells implementation in this study. (Color figure online) Raghavendra et al. 2018

Achieved from the MPQ-N-cells implementation, Figs. 5, 6 and 7 show further the results of the binary image transformation with the output of graphic contour lines for quantifying the six resulting segmented-patterns of various N-cells, i.e., the two segmented cells of mitochondrial antigens and intact mitochondria from Fig. 2(b)–(c), the two segmented MII cells from the column of Fig. 3(b) and the two segmented glioblastoma cells from the column of Fig. 4(b). Figures 5, 6 and 7(b) display their binary image representations in a logical array of 0 s and 1 s for computing the actual numbers of voxels within the segmented N-cells, while Figs. 5, 6 and 7(c) illustrate the output of graphic contour lines which sketch the bounding areas of the segmented N-cells with voxels for the measurement purpose.

Using the operation of region area calculation, Table 1 reports the quantitative results for the actual numbers of voxels within the six segmented-patterns of N-cells in Figs. 5, 6 and 7(a) {i.e., the bounding areas of the red/green regions within the two PD-related protein cells in Fig. 5(a), the bounding areas of the light green region within the two MII cells in Fig. 6(a) and the bounding areas of the green region within the two glioblastoma cells in Fig. 7(a)}. From Table 1, it can be observed that the image subject with N-cells of glioblastoma in the 2nd row of Fig. 7 is more progressive and aggressive with the number of 2846, spreading more extensively by 207.34% as compared to the other image subject with N-cells of glioblastoma in the 1st row of Fig. 7 with the number of 926 {(2846−926)/926 = 2.0734}; this would be useful for assessing the stages of disease quantitatively for patients with glioblastoma cancer in the disease diagnosis.

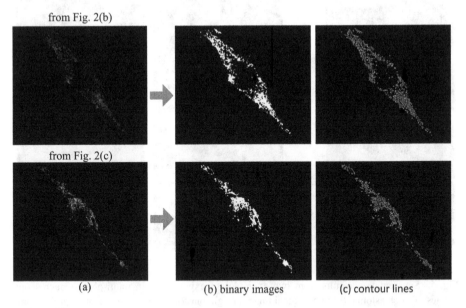

from Fig. 2(b)

from Fig. 2(c)

(a)   (b) binary images   (c) contour lines

Fig. 5. Results of the binary images of the segmented PD-related protein cells with the output of graphic contour lines from the PD-related protein image in the MPQ-N-cells implementation.

from the upper of Fig. 3(b)

from the lower of Fig. 3(b)

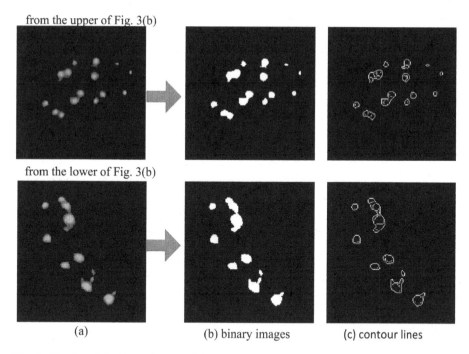

(a)   (b) binary images   (c) contour lines

Fig. 6. Results of the binary images of segmented MII cells with their contour line output from two examples of experiments on the PCDs-OPMD data in the MPQ-N-cells implementation.

from the upper in Fig. 4(b)

from the lower in Fig. 4(b)

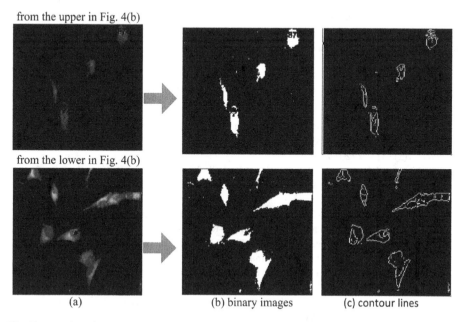

(a)   (b) binary images   (c) contour lines

Fig. 7. Results of the binary images of segmented glioblastoma cells with their contour line output from two examples of experiments in multi-photon microscopy images of glioblastoma in the MPQ-N-cells implementation.

Table 1. Quantitative results for measuring the six segmented patterns of N-cells related to diseases in Figs. 5, 6 and 7.

Measuring N-cells	PD-related protein	Figure 5 (a)	MII	Figure 6 (a)	glioblastoma	Figure 7 (a)
	Upper	Lower	Upper	Lower	Upper	Lower
#voxels in area of N-cells	6390	4306	860	1162	926	2846

4 Conclusion

In this study, without the prior knowledge of shapes of N-cells, the proposed MPQ-N-cells performs very well in the segmentation of irregular shapes of N-cells for measuring the patterns of N-cells related to PD, PCDs-OPMD and glioblastoma on the heterogeneous image datasets. The implementation results demonstrate the benefits of the design of the MPQ-N-cells, which is capable of providing simultaneously qualitative segmentation and quantitative measures of N-cells from the medical imaging. As the author is aware that experimental results in this study in measuring a variety of pathological N-cells with improved color visualization on the heterogeneous medical image datasets have not yet been reported in the literature in a comparable image cell-pattern segmentation scenario.

This study mainly focuses on the medical image data associated with the diseases of PD, PCDs-OPMD and glioblastoma cancer. Although the current proposed MPQ-N-cells has a limitation of the shortage of image data used in the implementation, this can be solved by implementing more medical images with access to big data. The future work will focus on presenting more results by conducting more experiments in big data sets, further develop the proposed approach to tracking the changes of cell for a longitudinal study on supporting the diagnoses of disease in medical imaging.

References

Ahmed, W., Fan, L.: Analyze physical design process using big data tool: hidden patterns, performance measures, predictive analysis and classifying logs. Int. J. Softw. Sci. Comput. Intell. **7**(2), 31–49 (2015)

Al-Kofahi, Y., Zaltsman, A., Graves, R., Marshall, W., Rusu, M.: A deep learning-based algorithm for 2-D cell segmentation in microscopy images. BMC Bioinformatics **19**(365), 1–11 (2018)

Bauer, S., Wiest, R., Nolte, L.-P., Reyes, M.: A survey of MRI-based medical image analysis for brain tumor studies. Phys. Med. Biol. **58**, R97–R129 (2013)

Bakas, S., et al.: Segmentation labels and radiomic features for the pre-operative scans of the TCGA-GBM collection. The Cancer Imaging Archive (2017)

Blumen, S.C., et al.: Cognitive impairment and reduced life span of oculopharyngeal muscular dystrophy homozygotes. J. Neurology **73**(8), 596–601 (2009)

Duyn, J.H.: The future of ultra-high field MRI and fMRI for study of the human brain. Neuroimage **62**, 1241–1248 (2012)

Deshmukh, B.S., Mankar, V.H.: Segmentation of microscopic images: A survey. In: International Conference Electronic Systems, Signal Processing and Computing Technologies, pp. 362–366 (2014)

Dzyubachyk, O., Niessen, W., Meijering, E.: Advanced level-set based multiple-cell segmentation and tracking in time-lapse fluorescence microscopy images. In: IEEE International Symposium on Biomedical Imaging: From Nano to Macro, pp. 185–188 (2008)

Egger, J., et al.: GBM volumetry using the 3D slicer medical image computing platform. Sci. rep. **1364**, 1–7 (2013)

Fereshtehnejad, S.M., Zeighami, Y., Dagher, A., Postuma, R.B.: Clinical criteria for subtyping Parkinson's disease: biomarkers and longitudinal progression. Brain **140**(7), 1959–1976 (2017)

Guo, P., Evans, A., Bhattacharya, P.: Nuclei segmentation for quantification of brain tumors in digital pathology images. Int. J. Softw. Sci. Comput. Intell. **10**, 36–49 (2018)

Guo, P.: A tissue-based biomarker model for predicting disease patterns. J. Knowl. Based Sys. **276**, 160–169 (2017)

Gui, L., Lisowski, R., Faundez, T., Huppi, P.S., Lazeyras, F., Kocher, M.: Morphology-driven automatic segmentation of MR images of the neonatal brain. Med. Image Anal. **16**, 1565–1579 (2012)

Gerard, I.J., Kersten-Oertel, M., Petrecca, K., Sirhan, D., Hall, J.A., Collins, D.L.: Brain shift in neuronavigation of brain tumours: a review. Med. Image Anal. **35**, 403–420 (2017)

Hortin, G.L., Carr, S.A., Anderson, N.L.: Introduction: advances in protein analysis for the clinical laboratory. Clin. Chem. **56**, 149–151 (2010)

Menze, B.H., et al.: The nultimodal brain tumor image segmentation benchmark (BRATS). IEEE Trans. Med. Imaging **34**, 1993–2024 (2015)

Murphy, R.F.: Communicating subcellular distributions. Cytometry, Part A **77A**, 686–692 (2010)

Otsu, N.: A threshold selection method from gray-level histograms. IEEE Trans. Syst. Man Cybern. **9**, 62–66 (1979)

Pärnamaa, T., Parts, L.: Accurate classification of protein subcellular localization from high-throughput microscopy images using deep learning. Gene Genomes Genet **7**(5), 1385–1392 (2017)

Rafael, R.C., Wood, R.E.: Digital Image Processing, 3rd edn. Prentice Hall, NJ (2008)

Raghavendra, A.J., et al.: Three-photon imaging using defect-induced photoluminescence in biocompatible ZnO nanoparticles. J. Nanomedicine **13**, 4283–4289 (2018)

Tohka, J.: Partial volume effect modeling for segmentation and tissue classification of brain magnetic resonance images: a review. World J Radiol. **11**, 855–864 (2014)

Tanti, G.K., Goswami, S.K.: SG2NA recruits DJ-1 and Akt into the mitochondria and membrane to protect cells from oxidative damage. Free Radical Biol. Med. **75**, 1–13 (2014)

Wang, J., et al.: Multi-atlas segmentation of subcortical brain structures via the AutoSeg software pipeline. Front. Neuroinform. **8**, 7 (2014). https://doi.org/10.3389/fninf.2014.00007

Spatiotemporal Statistical Model of Anatomical Landmarks on a Human Embryonic Brain

Aoi Shinjo[1]([✉])(ID), Atsushi Saito[1](ID), Tetsuya Takakuwa[2], Shigehito Yamada[2](ID),
Hidekata Hontani[3], Hiroshi Matsuzoe[3], Shoko Miyauchi[4], Ken'ichi Morooka[4],
and Akinobu Shimizu[1](ID)

[1] Tokyo University of Agriculture and Technology, Tokyo, Japan
s189227x@st.go.tuat.ac.jp, a-saito@go.tuat.ac.jp, simiz@cc.tuat.ac.jp
[2] Kyoto University, Kyoto, Japan
[3] Nagoya Institute of Technology, Aichi, Japan
[4] Kyushu University, Fukuoka, Japan

Abstract. We propose a new method for constructing a spatiotemporal statistical model of the distribution of anatomical landmarks (LMs) of a human embryo. This method exhibits potential for the quantitative assessment of the extent of anomalies and is important in the research of congenital malformations. However, a few of the LMs might not be observed at a specific developmental stage because large morphological deformations exist during the early stages of development. It is difficult for conventional statistical shape analysis methods to handle missing LMs in the training dataset. The basic concept of the proposed method is to conduct statistical analyses by predicting and completing the coordinates of the missing LMs. We demonstrated the proposed method in the context of spatiotemporal statistical modeling of 10 LMs on the brain surface using 37 embryonic subjects with Carnegie stages of 19–22. We conducted a comparative study of the spatiotemporal statistical models between four different prediction methods, and we found that deformable surface mapping was the best prediction method in terms of model generalization and specificity.

Keywords: Spatiotemporal analysis · Statistical model · Landmark · Embryo

1 Introduction

In human development, the embryonic stage (the third to ninth week of pregnancy) is a critical period for organ formation. It has been reported that malformation at birth occurs at a rate of 3% and causes up to one-quarter of all neonatal deaths [1,2]. Thus, a detailed analysis of embryos is important for the research of congenital malformations.

© Springer Nature Switzerland AG 2019
H. Greenspan et al. (Eds.): CLIP 2019/UNSURE 2019, LNCS 11840, pp. 94–103, 2019.
https://doi.org/10.1007/978-3-030-32689-0_10

A detailed three-dimensional (3D) shape analysis of early-stage embryos has been conducted in recent years. Embryo shape analysis not only facilitates understanding of developmental processes, but also serves as a basis for detecting abnormalities [3]. In [2], 3D images of embryos were reconstructed from digitized histological sections, and whole-body 3D digital atlases were developed for the quantitative analysis of development. Although the histology-based images offer sufficient resolution to visualize organ development, the image reconstruction process is extremely time-consuming. State-of-the-art magnetic resonance (MR) microscopy provides images with a spatial resolution of several 10 μm and is also useful for 3D embryo imaging. Using MR microscope images, morphometric analyses of various organs such as brain vesicles [3] and ocular organs [4] have been reported. However, these studies focused on typical temporal changes during development, and inter-individual shape variability is not thoroughly investigated.

The statistical models of anatomical structures such as landmarks (LMs) [5] and organ surfaces [6,7] have played a key role in revealing individual shape variability and are potentially useful for the quantitative assessment of the extent of anomalies [8]. Among the few studies of the statistical model for a human embryo, Saito et al. [9,10] developed a level set based statistical shape model of nested surfaces in a brain. These studies, however, only focused on a limited range of developmental stages, and the effect of developmental shape variability was not considered. To explain both individual and temporal shape variability, a spatiotemporal statistical model was proposed. Early studies of spatiotemporal statistical models are found in [11,12] where large deformation diffeomorphic metric mapping (LDDMM) was employed for heart and brain shape analysis. Kishimoto et al. [13] and Kasahara et al. [14] proposed a spatiotemporal statistical model for LMs of the eyeballs and brain surface of a human embryo, respectively. To calculate the temporally varying statistical model, they first constructed a statistical model for each developmental stage independently and then applied smooth interpolation between neighboring developmental stages. Alam et al. [15] employed expectation-maximization (EM) based weighted principal component analysis (PCA) with a temporal weight function to construct a spatiotemporal statistical shape model for brain deformation analysis. Similarly, a spatiotemporal statistical shape model of the pediatric liver was constructed in [16] using the weighted PCA with additional temporal regularization.

In this study, we propose a method to construct a spatiotemporal statistical model for semi-automatically extracted LMs on the brain surface of a human embryo that has not been addressed in previous literature. This is a challenging problem because there are a relatively large number of morphological changes, and a few LMs may appear and disappear during the early stages of development. Therefore, a few of the LMs are missing in the specific developmental stages and conventional spatiotemporal statistical analysis [13,14] cannot be applied. The algorithm proposed by Hufnagel et al. [17] deals with different numbers of LMs by performing shape analysis using probabilistic point correspondences. However, this method is not suitable when LMs have one-to-one point correspondences. To

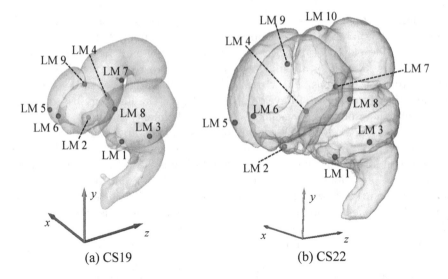

Fig. 1. LMs on the brain surface of human embryo (CS19 and CS22).

overcome this issue, we proposed methods to predict missing LMs using interpolation and extrapolation techniques, including deformable surface mapping
[18]. The proposed spatiotemporal statistical modeling method was applied to
10 anatomical LMs of a human embryo with the Carnegie stage (CS) of 19 to
22. Using 37 human embryos from the Kyoto Collection [19], different statistical models with four different prediction methods were compared based on the
generalization and the specificity of the model [20].

2   Methods

In this study, we focus on 10 LMs on the brain surface of human embryos, i.e.,
LM1–LM10 shown in Fig. 1, to be targets of statistical shape modeling. In our
dataset LM10 is missing for CS19 (Fig. 1(a)), but observed after CS20 (Fig. 1(b)).
Therefore, we apply a the spatiotemporal statistical analysis after the prediction
of the LM coordinate vectors. We explain the spatiotemporal statistical modeling
method in Sect. 2.1 followed by the LM prediction methods in Sect. 2.2.

2.1   Spatiotemporal Statistical Modeling

The model construction method is summarized in Fig. 2. First, the LM coordinates are vectorized, and all the subjects are mapped to the feature space
constructed by PCA. The statistics (mean and covariance) are then estimated
for each CS and are seamlessly interpolated between neighboring stages based
on the theory of information geometry [21]. Further details of the model construction method are described in the literature [13,14].

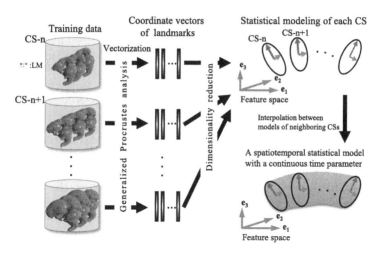

Fig. 2. Spatiotemporal statistical model construction method.

2.2 Prediction of the Missing Landmarks

This section describes a method to predict the location of LM10 of the embryo of CS19. We propose four prediction methods in this study:

- Averaging: Averaging the LM from the nearest CS
- LP(CCA): Linear prediction (LP) with canonical correlation analysis (CCA [22])
- LP(Nearest): LP with the nearest LM
- mSDM: Deformable surface mapping with modified self-organizing deformable model (mSDM) [18]

We describe the detail of the prediction algorithms below.

Averaging. This method estimates the coordinates of the missing LM by taking the average of the coordinates of the LMs over the subjects from the nearest CS. In other words, the average coordinates of LM10 in CS20 are used as the prediction of LM10 of CS19, which can be expressed as

$$Y_{19} = \overline{Y_{20}} \tag{1}$$

where Y_{19} is the estimated coordinate vector of LM10 at CS19, and $\overline{Y_{20}}$ represents the average coordinate vector of LM10 over all the training samples in CS20.

Linear Prediction (LP). LP is used to predict the location of LM10 from the other existing LMs in the same subject. The predictor is derived from the set of subjects from CS20–22 which have no missing LMs. Location of LM10 of CS19 in a given subject is predicted with the following equation:

$$Y_{19} = \left(AB^{-1}\right)^{\mathsf{T}} \left(X_{19} - \overline{X_{20\sim22}}\right) + \overline{Y_{20\sim22}} \tag{2}$$

where X_{19} is the coordinate vector of the LMs selected as the input of the prediction. $\overline{X}_{20\sim22}$ and $\overline{Y}_{20\sim22}$ represent the vectors of the average coordinates of the selected LMs and LM10 in CS20–22, respectively. Prediction matrices A and B are calculated using CCA as follows:

$$(A, B) = \underset{A,B}{\arg\max}\, A^{\mathsf{T}} S_{XY} B \quad s.t. \quad A^{\mathsf{T}} S_{XX} A = B^{\mathsf{T}} S_{YY} B = I \qquad (3)$$

where S_{XX}, S_{YY} and S_{XY} represent covariance matrices calculated for the predictor's input X and output Y obtained from training subjects in CS20–22.

In this study, we consider two different LPs according to the LMs used as the input: (i) LP using a LM with the highest correlation to the coordinate of LM10, which we denote as LP(CCA), and (ii) LP using the nearest LM, which we denote as LP(Nearest).

Deformable Surface Mapping (mSDM). We denote $\mathcal{M}$ as the surface of a subject with missing LMs (i.e., a subject of CS19) and $\mathcal{T}$ as the template shape on which all the LMs exist (i.e., a mean shape of the brains of CS20–CS22). Once the optimal transformation Φ^* that maps $\mathcal{M}$ to $\mathcal{T}$ has been calculated, the location of the missing LM Y_{19} on $\mathcal{M}$ is predicted using the following formula:

$$Y_{19} = (\Phi^*)^{-1} (Y') \qquad (4)$$

where Y' is the position of LM10 on the template shape $\mathcal{T}$.

Geometrical feature-preserving mapping constrained by LMs is adopted as the surface mapping method [18] where the optimal transformation Φ^* is calculated by solving the minimization problem:

$$\Phi^* = \underset{\Phi}{\arg\min} \left[w_f E_f \left(\Phi\left(\mathcal{M}\right), \mathcal{T} \right) + w_b E_b \left(\Phi\left(\mathcal{M}\right), \mathcal{T} \right) \right.$$
$$\left. + w_l E_l \left(\Phi\left(\mathcal{M}\right), \mathcal{T} \right) + w_g E_g \left(\mathcal{M}, \Phi\left(\mathcal{M}\right) \right) \right] \qquad (5)$$

where E_f, E_b, E_l, and E_g are the energy functions described in the next paragraph and w_f, w_b, w_l, and w_g are the weighting coefficients. Equation (5) is optimized according to Miyauchi et al. [18].

The first term E_f measures the fitness between the mapped brain surface $\Phi(\mathcal{M})$ and the mean shape $\mathcal{T}$:

$$E_f \left(\Phi\left(\mathcal{M}\right), \mathcal{T} \right) = \frac{1}{2} \left(\sum_{v \in \Gamma_T} \frac{H\left(v, \Phi\left(\mathcal{M}\right)\right)}{|\Gamma_T|} + \sum_{v \in \Gamma_M} \frac{H\left(\Phi\left(v\right), \mathcal{T}\right)}{|\Gamma_M|} \right) \qquad (6)$$

where Γ_T and Γ_M are the sets of vertices on $\mathcal{T}$ and $\mathcal{M}$, respectively, and $H\left(c, D\right)$ denotes the Euclidean distance between point c and the surface D. The second term E_b measures the frequency of foldover occurrence calculated by counting the number of folded patches in $\Phi(\mathcal{M})$ as

$$E_b(\Phi(\mathcal{M}), \mathcal{T}) = \sum_{p \in \mathcal{M}} B(\Phi(p), \mathcal{T})$$

$$\text{where} \quad B(\Phi(p), \mathcal{T}) = \begin{cases} 1 & (n(\Phi(p)) \cdot n(v'_{\mathcal{T}}) < \kappa) \\ 0 & (otherwise) \end{cases} \tag{7}$$

where $n(\Phi(p))$ is the normal of the mapped patch $\Phi(p)$ in $\Phi(\mathcal{M})$ and $v'_{\mathcal{T}}$ is the nearest vertex in $\mathcal{T}$ closest to $\Phi(p)$. In our experiment, the parameter κ is set to $\kappa = 0$. The third term E_l assesses the accuracy of mapping for the LM points:

$$E_l(\Phi(\mathcal{M}), \mathcal{T}) = \sum_{(u,v) \in \Lambda} \|\Phi(u) - v\| \tag{8}$$

where we denote Λ as the set of nine corresponding LM pairs in $\mathcal{M}$ and $\mathcal{T}$ existing in all the subjects. The last term E_g measures the geometrical feature preservation, which is formulated as

$$E_g(\mathcal{M}, \Phi(\mathcal{M})) = \mu E_{area}(\mathcal{M}, \Phi(\mathcal{M})) + (1 - \mu) E_{angle}(\mathcal{M}, \Phi(\mathcal{M})) \tag{9}$$

where μ is the weighting factor of the two distortion errors and is set to $\mu = 0.5$. Equation (9) enforces the mapping to preserve both areas and angles by measuring the distortion errors E_{area} and E_{angle} defined in Eqs. (10) and (11), respectively:

$$E_{area}(\mathcal{M}, \Phi(\mathcal{M})) = \sum_{p \in \mathcal{M}} \left| \frac{A(\Phi(p))}{A(\Phi(\mathcal{M}))} - \frac{A(p)}{A(\mathcal{M})} \right| \tag{10}$$

$$E_{angle}(\mathcal{M}, \Phi(\mathcal{M})) = \sum_{p \in \mathcal{M}} \sum_{d=0}^{2} |\theta(\Phi(p), d) - \theta(p, d)| \tag{11}$$

Here $A(p)$ and $\theta(p, d)$ denote the area and the d-th angle of the triangular patch p, respectively.

3   Experiments

The proposed method was demonstrated in the context of statistical shape modeling of the LMs of a human embryonic brain. This study was approved by the ethics committee of the Graduate School and Faculty of Medicine of Kyoto University (R0316, R0989) and the ethics committee of Tokyo University of Agriculture and Technology (No. 30-28). MR volumes were acquired by an MR microscope with a 2.35 T bore (40 cm) superconducting magnet (T1-weighted spin-echo sequences with a 100 ms repetition time and an echo time of 10–16 ms) [23]. Brain labels were manually delineated on the MR volumes using the FMRIB Software Library[TM] (ver. 4.1.9, Analysis Group, FMRIB, Oxford, UK) and Amira[TM] software (ver. 5.4.0, Visage Imaging, Berlin, Germany). We

Table 1. Comparison of the generalization and the specificity measures between four models. Brackets indicate the statistical significance ($** : p < 0.01$, $* : p < 0.05$).

Method	Generalization	Specificity
Averaging	0.3291	0.3395
LP(CCA)	0.3295	0.3790
LP(Nearest)	0.3373	0.3511
mSDM	**0.3252**	**0.3365**

defined LMs and control points on the brain surfaces semi-automatically and used them to perform the generalized Procrustes analysis involving translation, rotation, and scaling. We used 37 embryonic subjects with CS19 to 22. Brain surface meshes with 50,000 patches were constructed from the brain label volumes using MeshLab (http://www.meshlab.net/). After the prediction of the missing LMs, a spatiotemporal statistical model was constructed by the method [13,14].

A two-fold cross validation was carried out in this study. The performance of the proposed model was evaluated by both generalization and specificity [20] which are defined as Eqs. (12) and (13).

$$(\text{Generalization}) = \frac{1}{N\sqrt{w}} \sum_{n=1}^{N} \left\| Z_n - \hat{Z}_n \right\| \tag{12}$$

$$(\text{Specificity}) = \frac{1}{M\sqrt{w}} \sum_{m=1}^{M} \min_{n \in \{1,\dots,N\}} \left\| Z_n - R_m \right\| \tag{13}$$

Here Z_n and $\hat{Z}_n$ are the original and the reconstructed LM coordinate vectors of the n-th test subject, respectively. $\{R_1, \dots, R_M\}$ represents the M instances randomly generated from the model, and w denotes the number of LMs. Note that generalization and specificity were calculated only for the existing LMs. These evaluation indices represent errors and a smaller value is better.

Table 1 summarizes the performance indices of the four models with different prediction methods calculated in the cross validation study. Statistical hypothesis testing was conducted using paired-sample t-test and two-sample t-test for generalization and specificity, respectively, between the best performing method and the other three methods. The model using mSDM achieved the best generalization, but no statistically significant differences from the other three models were observed. However, mSDM showed the best specificity with statistically significant differences from all the other models. The results suggest that mSDM was the best prediction method out of the four methods for the spatiotemporal statistical modeling of the LMs.

Figure 3 compares the location of LM10 predicted by the four methods for a subject in CS19. In principle, except for mSDM, the predicted LMs are not

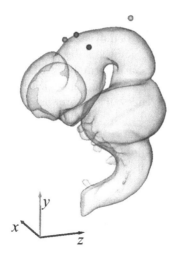

Fig. 3. Comparison of the four LM prediction methods for a subject of CS19. The purple, cyan, yellow, and red points show LM10 predicted by Averaging, LP(CCA), LP(Nearest), and mSDM, respectively. (Color figure online)

Table 2. Comparison of the prediction error between four prediction methods of LM10 in CS20. Brackets indicate the statistical significance (∗∗ : $p < 0.01$, ∗ : $p < 0.05$).

Method	Prediction error
Averaging	0.6902
LP(CCA)	1.069
LP(Nearest)	0.8612
mSDM	**0.4887**

necessarily in contact with the brain surface. On the other hand, the LM predicted by mSDM was on the brain surface and showed visually plausible results.

To quantitatively evaluate the accuracy of prediction, we measured the prediction error of LM10 using CS20 where the true location of LM10 is known. Table 2 summarizes the average prediction error obtained by the four prediction methods. The method mSDM achieved the lowest prediction error with statistically significant differences when compared to the other methods. This is consistent with the result in Table 1, and it suggested that reducing the prediction error is important in improving the performance of the spatiotemporal statistical model.

4   Conclusion

In this paper, we compared four methods for constructing spatiotemporal statistical models of LMs for organogenesis development. The effectiveness of the best performing method was demonstrated in the context of statistical shape modeling of the brain of a human embryo. Missing LMs were completed by the proposed prediction algorithms for the subsequent statistical analysis process. The prediction method based on deformable surface mapping performed best with respect to model generalization and specificity. In the future, we will further demonstrate the effectiveness of the proposed methods by increasing the number of missing LMs. In addition, we will investigate the applicability of the state-of-the-art missing data completion algorithm [24] for LM prediction. We also plan to demonstrate the applicability of the proposed spatiotemporal statistical model for quantification of the degree of morphological abnormality in embryonic development.

Acknowledgments. This work was partly supported by MEXT/JSPS KAKENHI Grant Numbers JP26108002, JP18H03255 and JP19K20291.

References

1. Kameda, T., Yamada, S., Uwabe, C., Suganuma, N.: Digitization of clinical and epidemiological data from the Kyoto Collection of Human Embryos: maternal risk factors and embryonic malformations. Congenit. Anom. **52**(1), 48–54 (2012)
2. de Bakker, B.S., et al.: An interactive three-dimensional digital atlas and quantitative database of human development. Science **354**(6315), aag0053 (2016)
3. Nakashima, T., Hirose, A., Yamada, S., Uwabe, C., Kose, K., Takakuwa, T.: Morphometric analysis of the brain vesicles during the human embryonic period by magnetic resonance microscopic imaging. Congenit. Anom. **52**(1), 55–58 (2012)
4. Osaka, M., et al.: Positional changes of the ocular organs during craniofacial development. Anat. Rec. **300**(12), 2107–2114 (2017)
5. Cootes, T.F., Taylor, C.J., Cooper, D.H., Graham, J.: Active shape models-their training and application. Comput. Vis. Image Underst. **61**(1), 38–59 (1995)
6. Cremers, D., Rousson, M., Deriche, R.: A review of statistical approaches to level set segmentation: integrating color, texture, motion and shape. Int. J. Comput. Vis. **72**(2), 195–215 (2007). https://doi.org/10.1007/s11263-006-8711-1
7. Heimann, T., Meinzer, H.P.: Statistical shape models for 3D medical image segmentation: a review. Med. Image Anal. **13**(4), 543–563 (2009)
8. Dall'Asta, A., et al.: Quantitative analysis of fetal facial morphology using 3D ultrasound and statistical shape modeling: a feasibility study. Am. J. Obstet. Gynecol. **217**(1), 76.e1–76.e8 (2017)
9. Saito, A., Tsujikawa, M., Takakuwa, T., Yamada, S., Shimizu, A.: Statistical shape model of nested structures based on the level set. In: Descoteaux, M., Maier-Hein, L., Franz, A., Jannin, P., Collins, D.L., Duchesne, S. (eds.) MICCAI 2017. LNCS, vol. 10433, pp. 169–176. Springer, Cham (2017). https://doi.org/10.1007/978-3-319-66182-7_20
10. Saito, A., Tsujikawa, M., Takakuwa, T., Yamada, S., Shimizu, A.: Level set distribution model of nested structures using logarithmic transformation. Med. Image Anal. **56**, 1–10 (2019)
11. Mansi, T., et al.: A Statistical model of right ventricle in tetralogy of fallot for prediction of remodelling and therapy planning. In: Yang, G.-Z., Hawkes, D., Rueckert, D., Noble, A., Taylor, C. (eds.) MICCAI 2009. LNCS, vol. 5761, pp. 214–221. Springer, Heidelberg (2009). https://doi.org/10.1007/978-3-642-04268-3_27

12. Qiu, A., Albert, M., Younes, L., Miller, M.I.: Time sequence diffeomorphic metric mapping and parallel transport track time-dependent shape changes. Neuroimage **45**(1), S51–S60 (2009)
13. Kishimoto, M., et al.: A spatiotemporal statistical model for eyeballs of human embryos. IEICE Trans. Inf. Syst. **100**(7), 1505–1515 (2017)
14. Kasahara, K., et al.: A spatiotemporal statistical shape model of the brain surface during human embryonic development. Adv. Biomed. Eng. **7**, 146–155 (2018)
15. Alam, S., Kobashi, S., Nakano, R., Morimoto, M., Aikawa1, S., Shimizu, A.: Spatiotemporal statistical shape model construction for longitudinal brain deformation analysis using weighted PCA. In: Computer Assisted Radiology and Surgery (CARS 2016), vol. 11, p. S204 (2016)
16. Saito, A., et al.: Construction of a spatiotemporal statistical shape model of pediatric liver from cross-sectional data. In: Frangi, A.F., Schnabel, J.A., Davatzikos, C., Alberola-López, C., Fichtinger, G. (eds.) MICCAI 2018. LNCS, vol. 11071, pp. 676–683. Springer, Cham (2018). https://doi.org/10.1007/978-3-030-00934-2_75
17. Hufnagel, H., Pennec, X., Ehrhardt, J., Handels, H., Ayache, N.: Shape analysis using a point-based statistical shape model built on correspondence probabilities. In: Ayache, N., Ourselin, S., Maeder, A. (eds.) MICCAI 2007. LNCS, vol. 4791, pp. 959–967. Springer, Heidelberg (2007). https://doi.org/10.1007/978-3-540-75757-3_116
18. Miyauchi, S., Morooka, K., Tsuji, T., Miyagi, Y., Fukuda, T., Kurazume, R.: Fast modified Self-organizing Deformable Model: geometrical feature-preserving mapping of organ models onto target surfaces with various shapes and topologies. Comput. Methods Programs Biomed. **157**(4), 237–250 (2018)
19. Yamaguchi, Y., Yamada, S.: The Kyoto collection of human embryos and fetuses: history and recent advancements in modern methods. Cells Tissues Organs **205**, 314–319 (2018)
20. Styner, M.A., et al.: Evaluation of 3D correspondence methods for model building. In: Taylor, C., Noble, J.A. (eds.) IPMI 2003. LNCS, vol. 2732, pp. 63–75. Springer, Heidelberg (2003). https://doi.org/10.1007/978-3-540-45087-0_6
21. Ohara, A., Suda, N., Amari, S.-I.: Dualistic differential geometry of positive definite matrices and its applications to related problems. Linear Algebra Appl. **247**, 31–53 (1996)
22. Glahn, R.H.: Canonical correlation and its relationship to discriminant analysis and multiple regression. J. Atmos. Sci. **25**, 23–31 (1968)
23. Matsuda, Y., et al.: Imaging of a large collection of human embryo using a super-parallel MR microscope. Magn. Reson. Med. Sci. **6**(3), 139–146 (2007)
24. Yokota, T., Hontani, H.: Simultaneous tensor completion and denoising by noise inequality constrained convex optimization. In: IEEE CVPR, pp. 15669–15682 (2019)

Spaciousness Filters for Non-contrast CT Volume Segmentation of the Intestine Region for Emergency Ileus Diagnosis

Hirohisa Oda[1](✉), Kohei Nishio[1], Takayuki Kitasaka[2], Benjamin Villard[1], Hizuru Amano[3,4], Kosuke Chiba[3], Akinari Hinoki[3], Hiroo Uchida[3], Kojiro Suzuki[5], Hayato Itoh[1], Masahiro Oda[1], and Kensaku Mori[1,6,7]

[1] Graduate School of Informatics, Nagoya University, Nagoya, Japan
`hoda@mori.m.is.nagoya-u.ac.jp`
[2] School of Information Science, Aichi Institute of Technology, Nagoya, Japan
[3] Graduate School of Medicine, University of Tokyo, Tokyo, Japan
[4] Nagoya University Graduate School of Medicine, Nagoya, Japan
[5] Department of Radiology, Aichi Medical University, Nagakute, Japan
[6] Information Technology Center, Nagoya University, Nagoya, Japan
[7] Research Center for Medical Bigdata, National Institute of Informatics, Tokyo, Japan

Abstract. This paper proposes enhancement filters for shape-specific regions, based on radial structure tensor (RST) analysis, which we name "spaciousness filters". RST analysis can be used in a similar way to Hessian analysis for classifying intensity structures. However, RST is insufficient for enhancing regions having little contrast or non-typical morphology. Our proposed filters enhance such regions by extending the ray search scheme of RST analysis to work as a filter evaluating spaciousness. We show applications to the abdominal CT of ileus patients having specific shapes. The intestines (including small intestines) of those patients consist of air, liquid and feces portions, and are not contrast-enhanced by barium. Enhancement of liquid and walls play key roles in the sufficient segmentation of intestines and division between neighboring regions. Experimental results on 7 clinical cases showed that the proposed intestine segmentation method produced higher Dice score (0.68) than traditional RST analysis (0.44), even without specific refinement processes like machine-learning-based false positive reduction.

Keywords: Local intensity structure analysis · Small bowel segmentation · 3D intestine modeling

1 Introduction

Ileus and intestinal obstruction are conditions that require emergency diagnosis and operation. CT volumes are used by clinicians to locate and identify the intestinal obstructions point. However, manual tracing of the small intestine on

© Springer Nature Switzerland AG 2019
H. Greenspan et al. (Eds.): CLIP 2019/UNSURE 2019, LNCS 11840, pp. 104–114, 2019.
https://doi.org/10.1007/978-3-030-32689-0_11

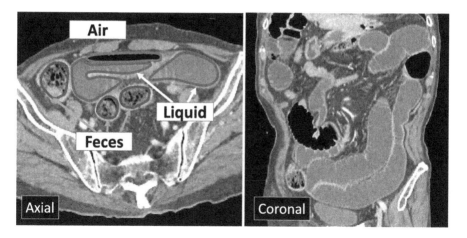

Fig. 1. CT volume of ileus patient. Contents of intestine consist of liquid, air and feces.

CT slice images is a time consuming and difficult task due to their complicated curves. Segmentation of intestines is desired for finding potential obstruction points. To the best of our knowledge, this work has only been carried out by our group. Automatic colon segmentation, as opposed to small intestine segmentation, has been widely studied for CT colonography [1,2]. Virtual cleansing [3] has also become a recent hot topic. Most of these studies do not focus on small intestines and require fecal tagging by contrast agent. Furthermore, injecting barium and waiting for hours to identify obstuction points is infeasible in emergency diagnosis.

Due to their success in segmentation applications, three-dimensional (3D) convolutional neural networks (CNN) could be used to segment small intestine region from CT volumes. However, this approach requires large numbers of annotated data in order to train the network such that it may achieve reasonable performance. Manual annotation of the small intestine is challenging process due to its anatomical structure, which is longer than the colon, as well as consists of winding structures that vary greatly. In order to segment these structures automatically, without the reliance on numerous pre-segmented data, we use a data-specific methodology by relying on filter-based approaches. Of these, Hessian analysis [4] is the most well-known method. Another approach is using a structure tensor or its extensions [5,6]. RST analysis is an extension of a structure tensor, that can be used in a way similar to Hessian analysis. The RST and Hessian analyses can be used for target structure enhancement filters (e.g. dark-tubular, bright-plate).

Both the RST and Hessian analyses enhance regions by respecting intensity differences around a target point. Intestines contains air, liquid and fecal matter (Fig. 1). Whilst intestine walls are contrast-enhanced, their gray values are very similar to liquid (Fig. 2). It is difficult to determine liquid as a dark-tubular structure (Fig. 3). To solve this problem, we propose to extend the ray search scheme

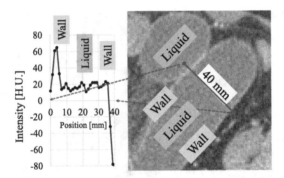

Fig. 2. Intensity profile on intestine. Liquid tentatively satisfies "dark-tubular," but walls are very thin and contrast is often low.

for RST computation, to also include shape information of surrounding spaces. We then apply our method to enhance walls and liquid regions of the intestines. Feces, located inside the intestine and colon walls, contain dark structures that represent air or other low density information. We segment these by using the morphologic dilation operation initialized from each individual dark structures. The dilation process iterates until it reaches the previously segmented walls.

Contributions of this paper are summarized as follows:

- (1) Extension of the ray search scheme for RST computation, which we name *spaciousness filters* (SF)
- (2) Parameter tuning of the SF for intestine walls (SF-walls) as well as for liquid (SF-Liquid)
- (3) Application of the SFs for non-contrast-enhanced intestine segmentation.

One advantage of our method is its reliance on the data at hand without the need for extensive annotated databases. In the experiments, we compare our proposed methods with conventional RST and Hessian analyses as a preliminary study using seven CT volumes. As the focus of this paper is to introduce SFs, we do not perform further refinement processes, e.g. shape model fitting or machine-learning-based false positive reduction.

2   Spaciousness Filters (SFs)

2.1   RST Analysis

Concept. Structure tensors (ST) are a common technique in image processing, e.g. Harris corner detection. Eigenvalues of the STs are non-negative and represent the extent to which intensities are changed along corresponding eigenvectors. The RST [7] is an improved structure tensor that produce even negative

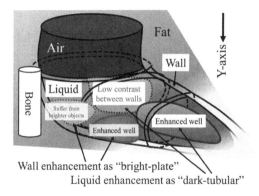

Fig. 3. Problems of conventional RST analysis for intestine enhancement. Common filters do not enhance liquid surrounded by walls which suffer from low gray values or walls with very high contrast between neighboring structures.

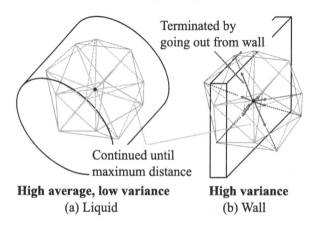

Fig. 4. Motivation of spaciousness filters (SFs). (a–b) Schema representing SF-Liquid and SF-Wall filters, respectively. Both regions are enhanced with respect to their characteristics of ray traveled distances. 12 vertices of regular icosahedron are drawn for simplicity, but 42 vertices are usually used including subdivisions of those vertices.

eigenvalues by introducing a radial search scheme. Rays travel to various directions, and each ray terminates when it encounters an edge-like point. This search scheme allows us to specify regions used for calculation of the tensor (Fig. 3).

Tensor. The RST $\boldsymbol{R}(\boldsymbol{x})$ at the point $\boldsymbol{x}$ is denoted by

$$\boldsymbol{R}(\boldsymbol{x}) = \sum_i \sum_j \alpha(\boldsymbol{x}, \boldsymbol{x}_{i,j}) \boldsymbol{g}(\boldsymbol{x}_{i,j}) \boldsymbol{r}_i^{\mathrm{T}} \tag{1}$$

where $\boldsymbol{x}_{i,j}$ represents a point in 3D coordinates (x, y, z) at j-th step on i-th ray ($i = 1, 2, \cdots, 42$ and $j = 1, 2, \cdots$). $\boldsymbol{g}(\boldsymbol{x}_{i,j})$ represent the intensity gradient around $\boldsymbol{x}_{i,j}$, and $\boldsymbol{r}_i$ represents the direction of the i-th ray. For each step on a ray, opacity $\alpha(\boldsymbol{x}_{i,j})$ $(0 \leq \alpha(\boldsymbol{x}_{i,j}) \leq 1)$ is computed as the absolute normalized intensity difference between $I(\boldsymbol{x})$ and $I(\boldsymbol{x}_{i,j})$.

Rays. Directions of rays should be distributed uniformly. For instance, as our data is in 3D, 42 rays can be defined as vertices of a sub-divided regular icosahedron. We use the termination condition $\mathcal{T} = 1$ in order to stop the individual rays, with respect to the accumulated opacity, such that

$$\mathcal{T} = \begin{cases} 1, & \text{if } \sum_{j=1,2,\ldots} \alpha(\boldsymbol{x}_{i,j}) \geq 1 \text{ or } |\boldsymbol{x}_{i,j} - \boldsymbol{x}| \geq R \\ 0, & \text{otherwise.} \end{cases} \tag{2}$$

The original point, or voxel of origin is represented by $\boldsymbol{x}$, and R is a user defined threshold, describing the maximum length of an individual ray. In our experiment we set $R = 15\,\text{mm}$.

Eigenvalue-Based Filters. Eigenvalues of $\boldsymbol{R}(\boldsymbol{x})$ behave similarly to those of a Hessian matrix. There exists bright or dark region enhancement functions for specific local intensity structures (blob-, line- or plate-like) [4,8], which are used to compare the eigenvalues of a Hessian matrix. These can be applied to RST without modification.

2.2   Spaciousness Evaluation for Targets

We introduce spaciousness filters (SFs) for our shape-specific target regions by modifying RST.

SF-Liquid. The length of the traveled rays are not only used for evaluating eigenvalues of the RST, but are also useful in identifying specific structures. As illustrated in Fig. 4(a), the liquid regions have the same constant intensity area, which can range from 10–40 mm in diameter. As such, if the distance traveled by the rays is high, we assume that the space around the target point $\boldsymbol{x}$ is large. Therefore, we developed our filter (SF-Liquid) to have a high response in the liquid region, as a function of traveled distance, such that

$$L(\boldsymbol{x}) = \frac{\mu(\mathcal{D}(\boldsymbol{x}))(J - \sigma(\mathcal{D}(\boldsymbol{x})))}{J^2}, \tag{3}$$

where $\mathcal{D}(\boldsymbol{x})$ represents the set of traveled distances of all rays from $\boldsymbol{x}$. $\mu(\mathcal{D}(\boldsymbol{x}))$ and $\sigma(\mathcal{D}(\boldsymbol{x}))$ represent the average and standard deviation of traveled distances in $\mathcal{D}$, respectively.

SF-Wall. In wall structures, some rays terminate very quickly while others travel for a longer period (Fig. 4(b)). As such, it is difficult to specify the range of mean distances, and thus, we only use the standard deviations, which are expected to be high. We developed this filter (SF-Wall) to have a high response in the wall region, as a function of traveled distance:

$$W(\boldsymbol{x}) = \frac{\sigma(\mathcal{D}(\boldsymbol{x}))}{J}. \tag{4}$$

Wall regions also satisfy the condition of bright "plate-like" structures of conventional RST analysis. We use this feature in our equation to assist in the conventional bright-plateness enhancement, as explained in Sect. 3.2.

3   Intestine Segmentation Method

3.1   Overview

Our proposed method requires an abdominal CT volume as input. We define the intensity of the volume I at a point $\boldsymbol{x} = (x, y, z)^{\mathrm{T}}$ as $I(\boldsymbol{x})$. We enhance the various structures, using our filters, in the following order: walls, contents of the intestines including liquid, feces and air. We then merged all the enhanced results to produce the final intestine segmentation.

3.2   Enhancement of Intestinal Anatomical Structures

Wall: Bright-Plateness and SF-Wall. Intestine walls have slightly higher values (around 50–100 Hounsfield Units (H.U.)) than liquid regions (around 0 H.U.). As previously mentioned, the bright-plateness filter does not respond well to such regions due to low contrast or neighboring bright objects. However, the SF-Wall is expected to enhance these regions, even in such conditions, as the SF-Wall focuses not only on intensity differences but as well on the termination of rays. The wall enhancement at $\boldsymbol{x}$ is obtained by

$$W(\boldsymbol{x}) = \max(\widehat{w}(\boldsymbol{x}), \widehat{p}(\boldsymbol{x})), \tag{5}$$

where $p(\boldsymbol{x})$ represents the bright-plateness filter's response [8] using conventional RST analysis. For comparing responses of different filters, we standardize the filter responses denoted by the symbol $\widehat{\ }$, which sets 95% of positive responses to be in the range $(0.0, 1.0]$ and all higher values as 1.0. We set $w_{\text{step}} = 1\,\text{mm}$ and $J = 5\,\text{mm}$ in our experiments.

Liquid: SF-Liquid. The SF-Liquid defined in Eq. (3) produces high responses in large flat regions. We use the SF-Liquid and the assumption that liquid is around 0 H.U. The response of our liquid enhancement filter is defined by

$$P(\boldsymbol{x}) = K(I(\boldsymbol{x}), c, w)\, L(\boldsymbol{x}), \tag{6}$$
$$K(v, c, w) = \max(0, \min(1/|v - c|, 1)), \tag{7}$$

where $k(v, c, w)$ $(0 \leq k(v, c, w) \leq 1)$ represents the triangular window function with center c and width w, which produces larger responses when value v is nearer to the center. In our experiments, we set $c = 0$ H.U. and $w = 50$ H.U. for focusing intensity range around liquid.

Feces: Dark-Blobs Segmentation. Fecal regions appear as random bright and dark regions in CT volumes. To remove them, we perform a dilation operation on each of the individual dark structures; which represent air or other low density information. In an initial step, we highlight dark structures using the conventional RST filter for dark blobs $\mathbf{B}(\boldsymbol{x})$. We define the responses for fecal regions by

$$F(\boldsymbol{x}) = D(\mathbf{B}(\boldsymbol{x}), b, d) \tag{8}$$

where $D(\mathbf{B}(\boldsymbol{x}), b, d)$ represents the dilation operation results of $\mathbf{B}(\boldsymbol{x})$ with width b which is performed until reaching regions which satisfy $m_W > 0$. We set $b = 5$ voxels in our experiments.

Air: Intensity. An intestine-like map is generated by integrating the maps for each of the components. The intestine enhancement value $m(\boldsymbol{x})$ at **x** is defined by

$$M(\boldsymbol{x}) = \left(1 - \widehat{W}(\boldsymbol{x})\right) \max\left(\widehat{A}(\boldsymbol{x}), \widehat{P}(\boldsymbol{x}), \widehat{F}(\boldsymbol{x})\right) \tag{9}$$

where $W(\boldsymbol{x}), P(\boldsymbol{x}), F(\boldsymbol{x})$ and $A(\boldsymbol{x})$ represent enhancement values of intestine walls, liquid, feces and air, respectively. The final segmentation of the intestines is obtained as the regions satisfying $M(\boldsymbol{x}) \geq 0.5$.

4   Experimental Results

Setup. Segmentation performances of the proposed method based on SFs are compared to the traditional RST or Hessian analyses. For RST and Hessian analyses, we used the dark-tubular filter [8] for enhancing liquid instead of the SF-Liquid. Walls were enhanced only by the bright-plateness filter. For fair comparison, we set $J = 20$ mm for RST's dark-tubular enhancement, which allows most rays to reach intestine walls from liquid. The programs are written in C++ and run on Windows 10.

Dataset. We utilized seven abdominal CT volumes of adult ileus patients scanned by Siemens or GE scanners, under IRB approval of (hidden institution). Seven axial slices of each CT volume have ground-truth labels for liquid, air and feces, which were manually traced by an expert. Pixel size for the CT volumes ranged from [0.625–0.789] mm, and slice thickness was 2 mm. We interpolated these CT volumes into 1 mm of isotropic resolution by cubic interpolation. For computing intensity gradients, Gaussian smoothing with 1.0 mm of standard deviation was performed as preprocessing.

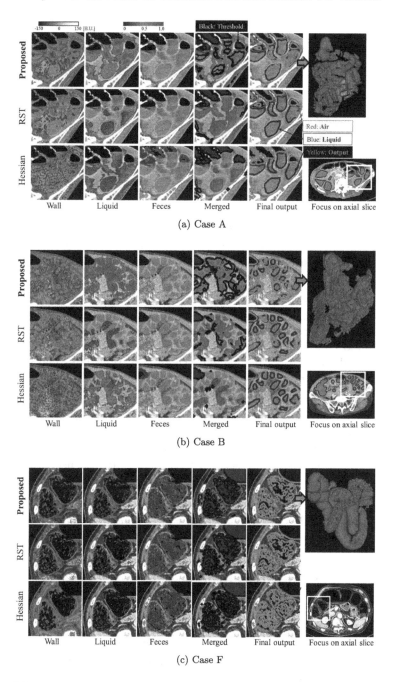

Fig. 5. Filter responses on CT axial slices and 3D rendering. (a) Example case (case A) having good liquid segmentation. (b) Example case (case B) showing poor liquid segmentation having connections between different regions and over-segmentation. (c) Example case (case F) containing feces. For better visualization of targets, 3D rendering is done by manually choosing various intestinal structures segmented using our method.

Table 1. Quantitative evaluation results between proposed method (Prop.), RST and Hessian (Hes.) analyses. Feces are evaluated only for cases C, F and G, which have ground-truth labels containing feces. **Bold** represents best performance.

Case	Dice score									# Connections per slice		
	Total			Liquid			Feces					
	Prop.	RST	Hes.	Prop.	RST	Hes.	Prop.	RST	Hes.	Prop.	RST	Hes.
A	**0.59**	0.41	0.50	**0.44**	0.06	0.07	N/A	N/A	N/A	**0.00**	**0.00**	1.00
B	**0.65**	0.19	0.23	**0.45**	0.05	0.11	0.00	**0.08**	0.01	1.29	**0.00**	1.14
C	**0.59**	0.38	0.33	**0.52**	0.28	0.11	0.12	**0.19**	0.13	**0.14**	0.86	1.14
D	**0.68**	0.36	0.10	**0.36**	0.32	0.02	**0.15**	0.13	0.12	1.00	0.57	**0.00**
E	**0.75**	0.55	0.48	**0.57**	0.37	0.16	N/A	N/A	N/A	**0.00**	1.43	1.29
F	0.74	0.72	**0.76**	0.08	**0.09**	0.09	**0.55**	0.50	0.34	**0.33**	1.17	1.33
G	**0.74**	0.43	0.29	**0.64**	0.40	0.28	**0.15**	0.10	0.07	0.14	0.57	**0.00**
Mean	**0.68**	0.43	0.38	**0.44**	0.22	0.12	0.19	**0.20**	0.13	**0.41**	0.66	0.84

Qualitative Evaluation. We visually compared responses obtained by our proposed method, RST and Hessian analyses for liquid, walls and feces. Examples of cases A and F, which contain much liquid and air, respectively, are shown in Fig. 5. 3D rendering is done by manually choosing various intestinal structures segmented using our method.

Quantitative Evaluation. The Dice score of each component (air, liquid, walls and feces) and their total value were compared on slices having ground-truth. We computed the Dice score between ground-truth and thresholded responses of the segmentation maps. Furthermore, we counted the connections between labels for our future application of tracking. These results are listed in Table 1.

Processing Time. Mean computational time of proposed method, RST and Hessian analyses was 6.7, 7.9 and 1.4 min per volume, respectively.

5   Discussions and Conclusions

Case A shown in Fig. 5(a) contains many liquid regions. It can be seen visually as well as in Table 1, that our method outperformed the other methods. The proposed method using SF-Wall performs qualitatively better in enhanced intestine walls, regardless of their low contrast. RST and Hessian analyses produced relatively strong responses to boundaries around air, however, intestine walls surrounding to fat or neighboring intestines did not have a strong response. Processing time of the proposed method was similar to RST analyses since there was no need to perform individual ray-searches using filters from conventional RST analysis.

A poor example of liquid enhancement is shown in Fig. 5(b), which produced over-segmentation and many connections. This is due to some intestine regions having small radii and low contrast. Furthermore, over-segmentation and connections occur across walls having low contrast, as this lack of contrast was insufficient for terminating the rays. Although we have tuned our spaciousness filters to perform better then other methods for cases where contrast is low, there exists the possibility to further extend our methodology to take into consideration the lack of contrast between walls and liquid.

Case F containing many feces is also shown in the second row of Fig. 5(c). Since SF-Wall produced high responses outside intestines, false positives outside intestines were suppressed by the proposed method. Segmentation of feces performed similarly by all methods, and only segmented parts of the regions as the bright parts of fecal matter were enhanced as well as the walls. It should be noted that feces in other cases were brighter than case F, which resulted in feces of those cases to be poorly segmented, as shown in Table 1.

In conclusion, we presented a novel methodology to segment intestines through a preliminary study which we validated on seven clinical cases. Our proposed SFs were useful for enhancing specific-shaped regions. Enhancing liquid in intestines and walls were efficiently performed for whole intestine segmentation. Furthermore, compared to deep learning methods which require large amounts of data and which are tailored to specific applications, our methodology is intrinsic and can be extended to broader applications. Our future work will consist of introducing more false positive reductions as well as an extension to the intestine tracking system.

Acknowledgements. Parts of this work were supported by the Hori Sciences & Arts Foundation, MEXT/JSPS KAKENHI (17H00867, 17K20099, 26108006, 26560255), JSPS Bilateral Joint Research Projects and AMED (19lk1010036h0001).

References

1. Wyatt, C., Ge, Y., Vining, D.: Automatic segmentation of the colon for virtual colonoscopy. Comput. Med. Imaging Graph. **24**(1), 1–9 (2000)
2. Tulum, G., Bolat, B., Osman, O.: A CAD of fully automated colonic polyp detection for contrasted and non-contrasted CT scans. Int. J. Comput. Assist. Radiol. Surg. **12**(4), 627–644 (2017). https://doi.org/10.1007/s11548-017-1521-9
3. Tachibana, R., et al.: Deep learning electronic cleansing for single- and dual-energy CT colonography. RadioGraphics **38**(7), 2034–2050 (2018). PMID: 30422761
4. Frangi, A.F., Niessen, W.J., Vincken, K.L., Viergever, M.A.: Multiscale vessel enhancement filtering. In: Wells, W.M., Colchester, A., Delp, S. (eds.) MICCAI 1998. LNCS, vol. 1496, pp. 130–137. Springer, Heidelberg (1998). https://doi.org/10.1007/BFb0056195
5. Arseneau, S., Cooperstock, J.R.: An asymmetrical diffusion framework for junction analysis. In: BMVC, pp. 689–698 (2006)
6. Arseneau, S., Cooperstock, J.R.: An improved representation of junctions through asymmetric tensor diffusion. In: Bebis, G., et al. (eds.) ISVC 2006. LNCS, vol. 4291, pp. 363–372. Springer, Heidelberg (2006). https://doi.org/10.1007/11919476_37

7. Wiemker, R., Klinder, T., Bergtholdt, M., Meetz, K., Carlsen, I.C., Bülow, T.: A radial structure tensor and its use for shape-encoding medical visualization of tubular and nodular structures. IEEE Trans. Visual Comput. Graphics **19**(3), 353–366 (2013)

8. Sato, Y., et al.: Tissue classification based on 3D local intensity structures for volume rendering. IEEE TVCG **6**(2), 160–180 (2000)

Recovering Physiological Changes in Nasal Anatomy with Confidence Estimates

Ayushi Sinha[1(✉)], Xingtong Liu[1], Masaru Ishii[2], Gregory D. Hager[1], and Russell H. Taylor[1]

[1] The Johns Hopkins University, Baltimore, USA
sinha@jhu.edu
[2] Johns Hopkins Medical Institutions, Baltimore, USA

Abstract. Between preoperative computed tomography (CT) image acquisition and endoscopic sinus surgery, the nasal cavity of a patient undergoes changes. These changes make it challenging for non-deformable vision-based registration algorithms to find accurate alignments between CT image and intraoperative video. Large alignment errors can lead to injuries to critical structures. In this paper, we present a deformable video-CT registration that deforms the *patient shape* extracted from CT according to statistics learned from population. We also associate confidence with regions of deformed shapes based on the location of matched video features. Experiments on both simulation and in vivo data produced $< 1\,\text{mm}$ errors (statistically significantly lower than prior work).

Keywords: Statistical shape models · Deformable registration · Confidence

1 Introduction

Since the step-by-step procedure for endoscopic sinus surgery (ESS) was first developed [14] in the early 1980s, interventions through the nasal cavities have become predominantly minimally invasive due to faster recovery times and reduced facial scarring. However, ESS comes with its own challenges. For instance, the 3D operating field is transformed into a 2D video display and the field of view (FOV) of the surgeon is limited to that of the endoscope. These can cause difficulty in estimating nearby anatomy that is not in the FOV of the endoscope. Knowledge of nearby anatomy is especially critical during surgeries through the nasal cavity since nasal cavities are small and complex with thin boundaries separating them from critical structures like the brain, eyes, carotid arteries, optic nerves, etc. Therefore, minimally invasive ESS through the nasal cavity requires a preoperative patient computed tomography (CT) scan, which is used by surgical navigation systems to orient surgeons with respect to critical anatomy.

© Springer Nature Switzerland AG 2019
H. Greenspan et al. (Eds.): CLIP 2019/UNSURE 2019, LNCS 11840, pp. 115–124, 2019.
https://doi.org/10.1007/978-3-030-32689-0_12

Several navigation systems have been introduced that register endoscopic views to preoperative patient CT image. Systems that use electromagnetic or optical trackers require markers to be attached to the endoscope, which can interfere with surgical workflow. Vision-based navigation systems, however, do not add any additional hardware to the surgical space. Many vision-based navigation systems compute rigid registrations between features from endoscopic video and CT image. The iterative closest point (ICP) algorithm [2] is a standard two-step registration algorithm that iterates between finding correspondences between feature sets and finding the transformation that best aligns the matched points until convergence. Several ICP variants have also been explored [21]. In addition to position, orientation [6,20], contours [4], and noise models [11,22] have been used to improve matches. However, patient anatomy undergoes change between CT image acquisition and surgery [12]. Patients are also administered decongestants before surgery which further modifies anatomy. Rigid registration methods have shown deterioration in performance in the presence of tissues that undergo change due to decongestants [15,16]. However, prior work has shown that principal component analysis (PCA) modes can capture the physiological changes that occur in the nasal cavity, i.e., the expanding and contracting of erectile tissues on the nasal turbinates [26]. Therefore, deformable variants of ICP that use PCA-based statistical shape models (SSMs) [9] to additionally solve for shape parameters have also been explored [13,27]. However, these methods compute registrations to the mean shape, deforming the mean shape to estimate patient, and do not take prior patient information into consideration. Further, they do not provide confidence measures on the estimated shape.

Our registration simultaneously computes video-CT registration and deforms *patient shape* using SSMs. We also estimate how errors in deformed patient shape estimation increase as distance from video features increases and provide confidence measures. We evaluate our method on simulated and in vivo data.

2   Method

The method in [27] is formulated according to the following likelihood function:

$$f_{\text{match\_def}}(\mathbf{x}, \mathbf{y}; \theta, \mathbf{s}, \bar{\mathbf{V}}, \mathbf{W}) = f_{\text{match}}(\mathbf{x}; T_{\text{ssm}}(\mathbf{y}, \mathbf{s}), \theta) \cdot f_{\text{shape}}(T_{\text{ssm}}(\mathbf{y}, \mathbf{s}); \mathbf{s}),$$

where f_{match} finds the oriented point $\mathbf{y} = (\mathbf{y_p}, \hat{\mathbf{y}}_{\mathbf{n}})$ on the current shape, ψ, that maximizes the likelihood of a match with oriented sample point $\mathbf{x} = (\mathbf{x_p}, \hat{\mathbf{x}}_{\mathbf{n}})$ from video, and f_{shape} is the likelihood of shape deformation. θ represents parameters of the non-deformable registration (i.e., rotation, R, translation, t, and scale, a), $\mathbf{s} = \{s\}$ represents the shape parameters, $\bar{\mathbf{V}}$ is the mean shape, $\mathbf{W}$ the weighted modes of variation, and T_{ssm} is the deformable transformation applied to $\bar{\mathbf{V}}$. f_{match} can be any likelihood-based registration objective, such as those presented in [3,5,6]. In this paper, we use the f_{match} defined in [6,27], which incorporates an anisotropic Gaussian noise model and an anisotropic Kent noise model to account for errors in position and orientation, respectively [6]. Assuming both position and orientation errors are zero-mean, i.i.d, f_{match} for each $\mathbf{x}$ transformed by a current similarity transform, $[a, \mathbf{R}, \mathbf{t}]$, is defined as [27]:

$$f_{\text{match}}(\mathbf{x}; \mathbf{y}, \boldsymbol{\Sigma}_\mathbf{x}, \boldsymbol{\Sigma}_\mathbf{y}, \kappa, \beta, \hat{\gamma}_1, \hat{\gamma}_2, a, \mathbf{R}, \mathbf{t}) = \frac{1}{\sqrt{(2\pi)^3|\boldsymbol{\Sigma}|} \cdot c(\kappa, \beta)}$$

$$\cdot e^{-\frac{1}{2}(\mathbf{y_p} - a\mathbf{R}\mathbf{x_p} - \mathbf{t})^\mathbf{T}\boldsymbol{\Sigma}^{-1}(\mathbf{y_p} - a\mathbf{R}\mathbf{x_p} - \mathbf{t}) - \kappa \hat{\mathbf{y}}_\mathbf{n}{}^\mathbf{T}\mathbf{R}\hat{\mathbf{x}}_\mathbf{n} + \beta\left((\hat{\gamma}_1{}^\mathbf{T}\mathbf{R}\hat{\mathbf{x}}_\mathbf{n})^2 - (\hat{\gamma}_2{}^\mathbf{T}\mathbf{R}\hat{\mathbf{x}}_\mathbf{n})^2\right)},$$

where $\boldsymbol{\Sigma} = \mathbf{R}\boldsymbol{\Sigma}_\mathbf{x}\mathbf{R}^\mathbf{T} + \boldsymbol{\Sigma}_\mathbf{y}$, $\boldsymbol{\Sigma}_\mathbf{x}$ and $\boldsymbol{\Sigma}_\mathbf{y}$ are the covariance matrices representing noise in $\mathbf{x}$ and $\mathbf{y}$, $\kappa = \frac{1}{\sigma^2}$ is the concentration parameter of orientation noise, σ is the standard deviation, and $\beta = e\frac{\kappa}{2}$ ($e \in [0, 1]$ is the eccentricity) controls the anisotropy of orientation noise along with $\hat{\gamma}_1$ and $\hat{\gamma}_2$, which are the major and minor axes of the elliptical level sets of the Kent distribution on the unit sphere [6, 18]. $\hat{\mathbf{y}}_\mathbf{n}$, $\hat{\gamma}_1$, $\hat{\gamma}_2$ are orthogonal. Similarly, assuming each vertex, $\mathbf{v} \in \mathbf{V}$, on a shape deforms independently and deformations are Gaussian distributed [23]:

$$f_{\text{shape}}(\mathbf{V}; \mathbf{s}) = \prod_{i=1}^{n_\mathbf{v}} f_{\text{vertex}}(\mathbf{v}_i; \mathbf{s}), \text{ where } f_{\text{vertex}}(\mathbf{v}; \mathbf{s}) = \prod_{i=1}^{n_\mathbf{m}} \frac{1}{(2\pi)^{3/2}}.e^{\frac{\|s_i\|_2^2}{2}}, \quad (1)$$

where $n_\mathbf{v}$ is the number of vertices in the shape and $n_\mathbf{m}$ is the number of PCA modes used to estimate deformation.

This formulation forces the mean shape to be the most likely shape [27] and cannot accommodate prior patient information. That is, in a generalized formulation for the exponent in Eq. 1, $e^{\frac{\|s_i - \mu_i\|_2^2}{2}}$, μ_i, which are the mode weights corresponding to the most likely shape, are simply set to 0, $\forall i$, since the mean shape produces $\mathbf{0}$ mode weights. This is a good assumption when patient CT is unavailable [25, 27]. However, if patient CT is available, then patient shape should be assumed to be the most likely shape. If patient shape, $\mathbf{V}^*$, is segmented such that it has correspondences with the mean shape [26, 28], μ can be computed by projecting the mean subtracted patient shape onto the SSM modes,

$$\mu_i = \mathbf{m}_i^\mathrm{T}(\mathbf{V}^* - \bar{\mathbf{V}})/\sqrt{\lambda_i},$$

where $\mathbf{m}$ and λ are the modes and mode weights of variation. $\mathbf{m}$ and λ can be obtained by performing PCA on a set of shapes with corresponding vertices [9]:

$$\boldsymbol{\Sigma}_{\text{SSM}} = \frac{1}{n_\mathbf{s}} \sum_{j=1}^{n_\mathbf{s}} (\mathbf{V}_j - \bar{\mathbf{V}})(\mathbf{V}_j - \bar{\mathbf{V}})^\mathrm{T} = [\mathbf{m}_1 \dots \mathbf{m}_{n_\mathbf{s}}] \begin{bmatrix} \lambda_1 & & \\ & \ddots & \\ & & \lambda_{n_\mathbf{s}} \end{bmatrix} [\mathbf{m}_1 \dots \mathbf{m}_{n_\mathbf{s}}]^\mathrm{T}.$$

Finally, the deformation applied to $\bar{\mathbf{V}}$ based on the current $\mathbf{s}$ is defined as

$$\mathrm{T}_{\text{ssm}}(\mathbf{y}_{\mathbf{p}_i}) = \sum_{j=1}^{3} \eta_i^{(j)} \mathrm{T}_{\text{ssm}}(\mathbf{v}_i^{(j)}), \text{ where } \mathrm{T}_{\text{ssm}}(\mathbf{v}_i) = \bar{\mathbf{v}}_i + \sum_{j=1}^{n_\mathbf{m}} s_j \mathbf{w}_j^{(i)},$$

$\eta_i^{(j)}$ are the 3 barycentric coordinates that define the position of $\mathbf{y}_i$ on a triangle on ψ, and $\mathbf{w}_i = \sqrt{\lambda_i}\mathbf{m}_i$ are the weighted modes of variation [27].

Finally, we associate confidence with regions of the estimated shape. We expect errors to be lower where sampled points are matched to the shape and higher as distance from these points increases since these areas are unobserved. To verify this, we associate per vertex errors with distance from the centroid of inlying matched points,

$$\mathbf{d}_i = \|\mathbf{v}_i - \mathbf{c}\|_2, \quad \text{where} \quad \mathbf{c} = \frac{1}{n_{\text{inliers}}} \sum_{i=1}^{n_{\text{inliers}}} \mathbf{y}_i,$$

and model our confidence based on observations in simulation. n_{inliers} is the number of inlying matched points.

3   Experiments and Analysis

Since our method initializes the shape estimation problem closer to the optimal solution, we expect our registrations to *converge faster* and produce *lower mean errors* since it is less likely for our optimization to converge to a non-optimal solution. To verify these expectations, we evaluate our method on simulated and in vivo data. All experiments are run on a 3.4 GHz Intel Core i7 CPU, 16 GB RAM.

3.1   Simulated Data

We perform a leave-one-out experiment using right nasal cavity meshes from a 53 CT dataset [1,7,8,10]. The left-out shape is perturbed to simulate a patient with modified anatomy. Points are sampled from regions of the perturbed left-out shape that would be visible to an endoscope (Fig. 3A). Position noise with $\sigma = 1 \times 1 \, \text{mm}^2$ in plane and 2 mm out of plane (i.e., $1 \times 1 \times 2 \, \text{mm}^3$) and orientation noise with $\sigma = 10°$ and $e = 0.5$ are added to the sampled points. Offsets in intervals $[0, 10]$ mm and $[0, 10]°$ are applied to the sample positions and orientations, respectively. The perturbed left-out shape is estimated using our method, i.e., with μ set to weights from the original left-out shape, and using prior work, i.e., with $\mu = \mathbf{0}$. Estimation of $\mathbf{s}$ is constrained to $[-3, 3]$ standard deviations. Both registrations are run with two noise assumptions: first, assuming the noise in the samples is known, and second, assuming the noise is unknown and initializing the noise estimates to $2 \times 2 \times 4 \, \text{mm}^3$ and $20°$ ($e = 0.5$) for position and orientation, respectively. To evaluate our results, we first compute the total registration error (tRE) by computing the Hausdorff distance (HD) between the deformed left-out shape and the estimated shape transformed to the coordinate frame of the registered sample points. Next, we compute the total shape error (tSE) by computing the HD between the two shapes in the same coordinate frame.

In both cases, we observed statistically significant[1] decrease in errors when registration is initialized to patient weights, with errors lower when noise is known (Fig. 1A and B) compared to when noise is unknown (Fig. 2A and B).

---

[1] All statistical significance figures reported in this paper are evaluated using the paired-sample Student's t-test and indicate $p < 0.001$.

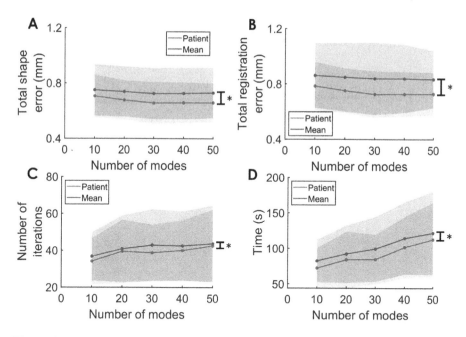

Fig. 1. Simulation experiment with known noise shows statistically significant (indicated by *) decrease in (A) tSE, (B) tRE, (C) number of iterations, and (D) runtime when registration is initialized to patient shape (green) rather than mean shape (red). (Color figure online)

We also observe that there is a statistically significant decrease in the number of iterations required for convergence, which also leads to decrease in runtime. Although there is a bigger decrease in number of iterations and runtime for convergence with known noise (Fig. 1C and D), results with unknown noise (Fig. 2C and D) show that for similar number of iterations and runtime, we achieve lower errors when registration is initialized to patient shape. Our current CPU implementation is embarrassingly parallelizable and can be further optimized to improve runtime.

We also observe, as expected, that shape estimation errors are lower where correspondences to sample points are found (Fig. 3B). Per vertex tSE shows little change near the centroid of the matched points, but quickly increases away from it (Fig. 4A). Therefore, we model our confidence in shape estimation as an exponential decay as distance from matched points increases. Figure 4B shows an estimated left-out shape from the experiment with unknown noise with ground truth errors, while Fig. 4C shows our estimated confidence in shape estimation.

3.2 In Vivo Data

Our clinical evaluation was performed on anonymized endoscopic videos of the nasal cavity collected from 4 consenting patients under an IRB approved

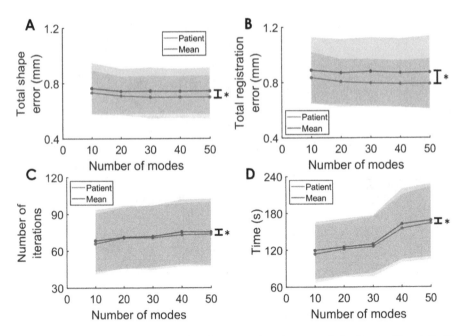

Fig. 2. Simulation experiment with unknown noise shows statistically significant (indicated by *) decrease in (A) tSE, (B) tRE, (C) number of iterations, and (D) runtime when registration is initialized to patient shape (green) rather than mean shape (red). (Color figure online)

protocol. These videos were used to train a self-supervised depth-estimation network that leverages established multi-view stereo methods like structure from motion (SfM) for learning [17]. This method produces dense and accurate point clouds from single frames of monocular endoscopic videos. Reconstructions from nearby frames were aligned using relative camera motion to produce dense reconstructions covering large areas in the nasal cavities. 3000 randomly sampled points from 14 such reconstructions were deformably registered both to the mean shape and the patient shape assuming noise with $\sigma = 1 \times 1 \times 2\,\text{mm}^3$ and $30°$ ($e = 0.5$) in position and orientation, respectively. The SSM used is pre-built using our 53 CT dataset and does not include CTs from any of the patients scoped for clinical evaluation. Rigid registrations to the respective patient shapes with the same parameters were also computed for comparison [6]. All registrations were manually initialized.

Since in vivo data lacks ground truth, we evaluate our registration using residual errors between matches computed by the registration. However, residual error can be misleading since it does not take into consideration the orientations of matched points. Therefore, we also report registration confidence based on the agreement in the orientations of corresponding points. [27] showed that registration confidence decreased with increasing chi-square CDF values, p, computed

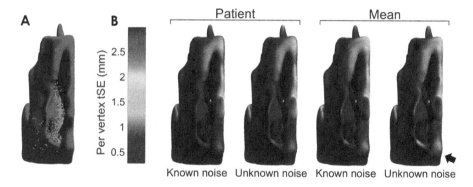

Fig. 3. (A) Right nasal cavity mesh with an example of points (yellow) sampled from the inferior turbinate, lateral and septal walls, and cavity floor - regions visible to an endoscope when entering the cavity. (B) Mean tSE over registrations (from L-R) initialized at patient shape and mean shape, with known and unknown noise each, and run with 50 modes plotted on the mean shape. Shape estimation errors are higher away from matched points as well as when mean shape is used for initialization (arrow). (Color figure online)

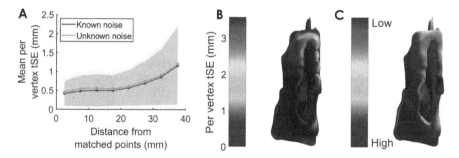

Fig. 4. (A) Trend in shape estimation errors as distance from matched points increases. (B) Ground truth shape estimation errors on an estimated left-out shape and (C) our estimated confidence. Blue indicates high confidence while red indicates low confidence. (Color figure online)

using orientation agreement scores. For simplicity, we show increasing confidence with increasing $q = 1 - p$.

Both deformable registration methods produced statistically significant improvements over rigid registration to patient shape, which produced a mean residual error of $0.7\,(\pm 0.26)$ mm. Residual errors between deformable registration initialized at mean shape and initialized at patient shape produced the same residual error of $0.44\,(\pm 0.14)$ mm. However, confidence in registration using orientation agreement was higher when initialized to patient shape (Fig. 5A), implying that our method produced better alignment. We are also able to visualize confidence in estimated shapes. Confidence in estimated Patient 2 is shown in Fig. 5B along with the alignment that produced the estimated shape (Fig. 5C and D).

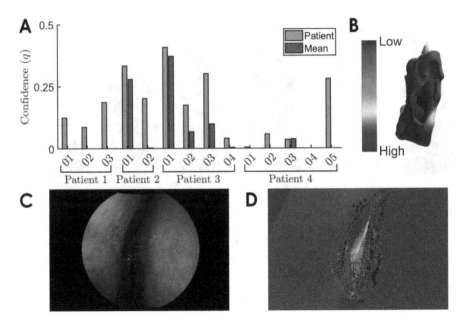

Fig. 5. (A) Confidence based on orientation agreement plotted for registrations computed with reconstructions from different video sequences. Initializations at patient shape (green) produce higher confidence in registration, only showing no confidence for sequences 01 and 04 from Patient 4. Several registrations initialized at mean shape (red) show no confidence. (B) Deformed patient 2 with confidence estimates when aligned with features extracted from (C) video sequence 02. (D) Points (red with blue normals) overlayed on the deformed shape (gray). (Color figure online)

4   Discussion and Future Work

In this work, we show that we can deformably register endoscopic videos to patient CT using PCA modes to deform *patient shape*. This method produces statistically significant improvements in registration errors as well as iterations and runtime to convergence compared to prior PCA-based deformable registration methods [24]. We believe that these results bring us a step closer to providing accurate patient-specific navigation during endoscopic sinus procedures without using any external tools like electromagnetic or optical trackers.

We did not compare our method to other prior registration methods like coherent point drift (CPD) due to memory limitations [19]. CPD computes a $n_{\mathbf{v}} \times n_{\mathbf{v}}$ matrix which is stored in memory, resulting in large memory overhead even for medium sized meshes. Our method does not suffer from such limitations. Further, we expect our method to perform as well [24] or better since CPD only deforms the parts of meshes where sample points are matched which can result in unnatural deformations in the mesh. Since our method is driven by statistics learned from population, it is much less likely for our method to produce unnatural deformations. Our method also computes confidence falloff in estimated shapes as distance from registered feature points increases. Providing this information during surgical navigation is critical since it allows surgeons to modulate their trust in the navigation system.

In the future, we will analytically evaluate the uncertainty in different regions of the estimated shape and improve the runtime of our algorithm. We are also working on building SSMs from a larger population in order to better capture the extent of variations in the nasal cavity. Another goal we hope to work towards is automating registration initialization so our method can be seamlessly integrated into the surgical navigation workflow. Finally, we would like to emphasize that our method can enable highly accurate navigation and reduce risk of damage to critical structures towards the start of a procedure. We hope that future work that can account for non-physiological changes that occur during surgery can be integrated with our method to enable accurate navigation throughout endoscopic sinus procedures.

Acknowledgment. This work was funded by the Johns Hopkins University (JHU) Provost's Postdoctoral Fellowship and other JHU internal funds. We would also like to thank Seth D. Billings for his invaluable feedback.

References

1. Beichel, R.R., et al.: Data from QIN-HEADNECK. The Cancer Imaging Archive (2015)
2. Besl, P.J., McKay, N.D.: A method for registration of 3-D shapes. IEEE Trans. Pattern Anal. Mach. Intell. **14**(2), 239–256 (1992)
3. Billings, S.D., Boctor, E.M., Taylor, R.H.: Iterative most-likely point registration (IMLP): a robust algorithm for computing optimal shape alignment. PLoS ONE **10**(3), 1–45 (2015)
4. Billings, S.D., et al.: Anatomically constrained video-CT registration via the V-IMLOP algorithm. In: Ourselin, S., Joskowicz, L., Sabuncu, M.R., Unal, G., Wells, W. (eds.) MICCAI 2016. LNCS, vol. 9902, pp. 133–141. Springer, Cham (2016). https://doi.org/10.1007/978-3-319-46726-9_16
5. Billings, S., Taylor, R.: Iterative most likely oriented point registration. In: Golland, P., Hata, N., Barillot, C., Hornegger, J., Howe, R. (eds.) MICCAI 2014. LNCS, vol. 8673, pp. 178–185. Springer, Cham (2014). https://doi.org/10.1007/978-3-319-10404-1_23
6. Billings, S.D., Taylor, R.H.: Generalized iterative most likely oriented-point (G-IMLOP) registration. Int. J. Comput. Assist. Radiol. Surg. **10**(8), 1213–1226 (2015)
7. Bosch, W.R., Straube, W.L., Matthews, J.W., Purdy, J.A.: Data from Head-Neck-Cetuximab. The Cancer Imaging Archive (2015)
8. Clark, K., et al.: The cancer imaging archive (TCIA): maintaining and operating a public information repository. J. Digit. Imaging **26**(6), 1045–1057 (2013)
9. Cootes, T.F., Taylor, C.J., Cooper, D.H., Graham, J.: Active shape models - their training and application. Comput. Vis. Image Underst. **61**, 38–59 (1995)
10. Fedorov, A., et al.: DICOM for quantitative imaging biomarker development: a standards based approach to sharing clinical data and structured PET/CT analysis results in head and neck cancer research. PeerJ **4**, e2057 (2016)

11. Granger, S., Pennec, X.: Multi-scale EM-ICP: a fast and robust approach for surface registration. In: Heyden, A., Sparr, G., Nielsen, M., Johansen, P. (eds.) ECCV 2002. LNCS, vol. 2353, pp. 418–432. Springer, Heidelberg (2002). https://doi.org/10.1007/3-540-47979-1_28

12. Hasegawa, M., Kern, E.B.: The human nasal cycle. Mayo Clin. Proc. **52**(1), 28–34 (1977)

13. Hufnagel, H., Pennec, X., Ehrhardt, J., Ayache, N., Handels, H.: Computation of a probabilistic statistical shape model in a maximum-a-posteriori framework. Methods Inf. Med. **48**(04), 314–319 (2009)

14. Kennedy, D.W.: Functional endoscopic sinus surgery. Technique. Arch. Otolaryngol. **111**(10), 643–649 (1985). (Chicago, Ill.: 1960)

15. Leonard, S., et al.: Evaluation and stability analysis of video-based navigation system for functional endoscopic sinus surgery on in vivo clinical data. IEEE Trans. Med. Imaging **37**(10), 2185–2195 (2018)

16. Leonard, S., Reiter, A., Sinha, A., Ishii, M., Taylor, R.H., Hager, G.D.: Image-based navigation for functional endoscopic sinus surgery using structure from motion. In: Proceedings SPIE Medical Imaging, vol. 9784, pp. 97840V–97840V-7 (2016)

17. Liu, X., et al.: Self-supervised learning for dense depth estimation in monocular endoscopy. In: Stoyanov, D., et al. (eds.) CARE/CLIP/OR 2.0/ISIC -2018. LNCS, vol. 11041, pp. 128–138. Springer, Cham (2018). https://doi.org/10.1007/978-3-030-01201-4_15

18. Mardia, K.V., Jupp, P.E.: Directional Statistics. Wiley Series in Probability and Statistics, pp. 1–432. Wiley, Hoboken (2008)

19. Myronenko, A., Song, X.: Point set registration: coherent point drift. IEEE Trans. Pattern Anal. Mach. Intell. **32**(12), 2262–2275 (2010)

20. Pulli, K.: Multiview registration for large data sets. In: Proceedings 2nd International Conference on 3-D Digital Imaging and Modeling, pp. 160–168 (1999)

21. Rusinkiewicz, S., Levoy, M.: Efficient variants of the ICP algorithm. In: Proceedings 3rd International Conference on 3-D Digital Imaging and Modeling, pp. 145–152 (2001)

22. Segal, A., Haehnel, D., Thrun, S.: Generalized-ICP. In: Proceedings Robotics: Science & Systems (2009)

23. Sinha, A.: Deformable registration using shape statistics with applications in sinus surgery. Ph.D. thesis, The Johns Hopkins University (2018)

24. Sinha, A., et al.: The deformable most-likely-point paradigm. Med. Image Anal. **55**, 148–164 (2019)

25. Sinha, A., Ishii, M., Hager, G.D., Taylor, R.H.: Endoscopic navigation in the clinic: registration in the absence of preoperative imaging. Int. J. Comput. Assist. Radiol. Surg. **14**, 12 (2019). IJCARS-MICCAI 2018

26. Sinha, A., Leonard, S., Reiter, A., Ishii, M., Taylor, R.H., Hager, G.D.: Automatic segmentation and statistical shape modeling of the paranasal sinuses to estimate natural variations. In: Proceedings SPIE Medical Imaging, vol. 9784, pp. 97840D–97840D-8 (2016)

27. Sinha, A., Liu, X., Reiter, A., Ishii, M., Hager, G.D., Taylor, R.H.: Endoscopic navigation in the absence of CT imaging. In: Frangi, A.F., Schnabel, J.A., Davatzikos, C., Alberola-López, C., Fichtinger, G. (eds.) MICCAI 2018. LNCS, vol. 11073, pp. 64–71. Springer, Cham (2018). https://doi.org/10.1007/978-3-030-00937-3_8

28. Sinha, A., Reiter, A., Leonard, S., Ishii, M., Hager, G.D., Taylor, R.H.: Simultaneous segmentation and correspondence improvement using statistical modes. In: Proceedings SPIE Medical Imaging, vol. 10133, pp. 101331B–101331B-8 (2017)

Synthesis of Medical Images Using GANs

Luise Middel[1]([✉]), Christoph Palm[2,3], and Marius Erdt[1,4]

[1] Fraunhofer Singapore, Singapore, Singapore
luise.middel@gmail.com
[2] Regensburg Medical Image Computing (ReMIC), Regensburg, Germany
[3] Ostbayerische Technische Hochschule Regensburg (OTH Regensburg),
Regensburg, Germany
[4] Nanyang Technological University (NTU), Singapore, Singapore
marius.erdt@fraunhofer.sg

Abstract. The success of artificial intelligence in medicine is based on the need for large amounts of high quality training data. Sharing of medical image data, however, is often restricted by laws such as doctor-patient confidentiality. Although there are publicly available medical datasets, their quality and quantity are often low. Moreover, datasets are often imbalanced and only represent a fraction of the images generated in hospitals or clinics and can thus usually only be used as training data for specific problems. The introduction of generative adversarial networks (GANs) provides a mean to generate artificial images by training two convolutional networks. This paper proposes a method which uses GANs trained on medical images in order to generate a large number of artificial images that could be used to train other artificial intelligence algorithms. This work is a first step towards alleviating data privacy concerns and being able to publicly share data that still contains a substantial amount of the information in the original private data. The method has been evaluated on several public datasets and quantitative and qualitative tests showing promising results.

Keywords: Medical images · Generative adversarial networks · Data privacy

1 Introduction

The diversity of images created within a hospital is enormous, varying in respect of patient, the depicted content and the used modality. Using artificial intelligence in order to perform classifications, registration or segmentation on the images can reduce the doctor's workload and improve the overall efficiency of hospitals and clinics. A successful implementation such as the classifier to detect skin melanomas [1] uses more than 100,000 images in order to achieve accurate results. However, getting access to such amounts of images is often only possible for large corporations and hospitals, as this information is sensitive cannot be

© Springer Nature Switzerland AG 2019
H. Greenspan et al. (Eds.): CLIP 2019/UNSURE 2019, LNCS 11840, pp. 125–134, 2019.
https://doi.org/10.1007/978-3-030-32689-0_13

shared with the public due to doctor-patient confidentiality. Generative adversarial networks (GANs) could be applied on large datasets within hospitals in order to create synthetic data that can be shared with the public. The following enumeration describing Fig. 1 introduces a possible solution overcome the limitations of data privacy.

1. Medical images (X-rays, MRIs, CTs) are generated in the hospital. The images are then used for their original purpose (patient diagnosis, surgery planning, etc).
2. The images cannot be uploaded onto a cloud to be shared with the public due to data privacy regulations.
3. The same images are saved on the hospital server (not accessible by the public). Any authorized employee can start a user application to train a model that represents the statistical information of the images. A neural network is depicted in order to represent any deep learning model that may be used in this step. It converts the input data into statistical information.
4. The model generates images that show a great variety of the features in the model's input images while still showing the same basic object. It can be used to create any number of artificial images.
5. The generated images or the trained model can then be uploaded into the cloud and be shared with the public without concern for data privacy issues. In order to avoid sharing of generated data too similar to any of the original images, only a subset of the generated data with a certain distance to the originals could be shared.

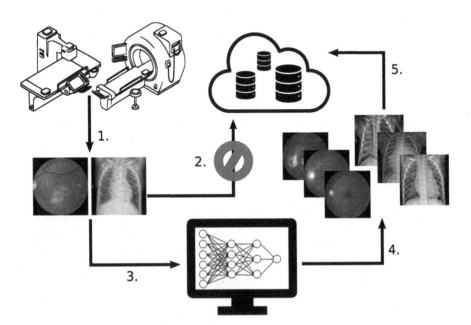

Fig. 1. Concept on how to make medical images publicly available. Image source by arrow number: 1: [2], 3, 5: [3,4]

A broader availability of such images creates the possibility of collecting more ideas and research results about solving complicated and common medical problems.

2   Background and Related Work

GANs were first introduced in [5] and are based on an adversarial principle. There are two players: the generator (G) and the discriminator (D). G is a neural network that generates images from a noise vector, whereas D is a neural network that tries to distinct between original image or generated image. The goal is to find the Nash equilibrium, where neither G nor D can change in order to improve the results. The process can be written as a minimax game:

$$\min_{G} \max_{D} V(D, G) = E_{x \sim p_{data}(x)}[\log D(x)] + E_{z \sim p_z(z)}[\log(1 - D(G(z)))] \quad (1)$$

GANs are of great interest in medicine due to the necessity of unsupervised learning, as labeled data is time consuming and rare. Examples of successful GAN applications for medical images are [6] which improves segmentation performance when introducing data variety into a brain-tumor dataset, [7] shows great promise with an implementation of a progressive GAN in order to generate realistic mammography images of a resolution of up to 1280×1024. [8] synthesizes realistic-looking retinal images working with only a small dataset of as few as 10 training examples of annotated binary vessels and applying style transfer.

3   Proposed Model

WGAN-gradient penalty (WGAN-GP) [9] provides a method to create sharp, realistic looking images without being prone to mode collapse and training instability due to unbalanced D and G. WGAN-GP is an improvement over the prior WGAN model [10] it is based on. The Earth mover distance (or Wasserstein-1-distance) is used to calculate the cost of transporting the estimated data distribution into the real data distribution using the Kantorovich-Rubinstein duality. In order to solve this equation and find the smallest loss, the functions used within must be 1-Lipschitz. This is achieved by introducing the gradient penalty that penalizes every function if it strays from the target norm value of 1. The discriminator loss can be written as:

$$L = \underbrace{E_{\bar{x} \sim P_g}[D(\bar{x})] - E_{x \sim P_r}[D(x)]}_{\text{original discriminator loss}} + \underbrace{\lambda \, E_{\hat{x} \sim P_{\hat{x}}}[(\|\nabla_{\hat{x}} D(\hat{x})\|_2 - 1)^2]}_{\text{gradient penalty}} \quad (2)$$

Where the first term represents the regular discriminator loss and the second one the gradient penalty multiplied with a fixed *penalty coefficient* λ. $\hat{x} \sim P_{\hat{x}}$ represents randomly sampled data points between the data distribution P_r and the generator distribution P_g.

The WGAN-GP implemented for this paper is based on images of size $128 \times 128 \times 3$. G and D are both convolutional neural networks with characteristics as specified in [9]. The input for G is a random noise vector of size 100 which is then upsampled by 6 transposed convolutional layers using 512, 256, 126, 64 and 32 different filters with a stride of 2. The input for D is an image of size $128 \times 128 \times 3$ which is either real or generated, and downsamples it with the use of four convolutional layers with 64, 128, 256 and 512 filters each.

Hyperparameters (learning rate, batch size and kernel size) were chosen on a trial and error basis, since there are currently no standard values that work well for all datasets. Values of hyperparameters with overall good visual results were achieved with a learning rate of 0.0002, a batch size of 32 and a kernel size of 5.

The models were trained for 500 epochs (chest X-rays with all images, pneumonia, non-pneumonia) and 10,000 epochs (chest with 115 images, AMD, non-AMD) respectively. See Sect. 4 for dataset name references. The number of epochs may still be increased, but the chosen amount showed a stabilization of the discriminator and generator loss.

4   Data

The evaluation is based on WGAN-GP models trained on three different two-dimensional datasets. All images are resized to RGB images of size $128 \times 128 \times 3$.

Two datasets were created from the **NIH chest X-ray dataset** [11]. The first one (referred to as **chest-all**) consists of 5606 chest X-rays of size 1024×1024 by multiple patients (Fig. 2a). The second one consists of 115 randomly chosen images (further referred to as **chest-115**).

The **Kaggle Pneumonia dataset** [4] shows chest X-rays of pediatric patients and can be split into 3,875 images of patients with pneumonia (referred to as **pneumonia**, Fig. 2b) and 1,341 patients without pathological findings (referred to as **non-pneumonia**, Fig. 2c). The significant difference to the previous dataset is that the images are less heterogeneous. However, the images are of different sizes which is why the resizing process creates slight distortions. This will be ignored as the evaluation is based on the original resized images. For real-life scenarios this should be avoided.

Lastly, the **age-related macular degeneration (AMD) dataset** [3] shows fundus photographs (photograph of the rear of the eye) of size 2124×2056

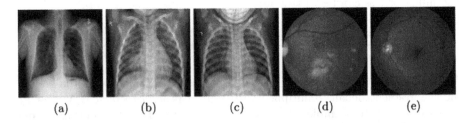

| (a) | (b) | (c) | (d) | (e) |

Fig. 2. Original dataset examples. (a) Chest, (b) Pneumonia, (c) Non-pneumonia, (d) AMD, (e) Non-AMD

pixels. It can be further divided into 89 images with AMD diagnosis (referred to as **AMD**, Fig. 2d) and 311 images showing normal maculae (referred to as **non-AMD**, Fig. 2e).

5   Evaluation Methods

The methods below are used to compare the results of the generated images and how the characteristics of the datasets influence the results.

5.1   Fréchet Inception Distance

The Fréchet Inception Distance (FID) [12] uses an Inception Net trained on ImageNet to measure the distance between the real data distribution and the generated data distribution with the Fréchet distance. A low FID value corresponds to a small distance between the data distributions which should correspond to good visual results.

5.2   Structural Similarity and Mean Squared Error

SSIM [13] is a metric to compare two images, based on the human visual system. This is commonly used when evaluating image compression. It is made up of three local comparisons: luminance, contrast and structure. The combination of the three features returns a value between -1 and 1, where 1 indicates very similar images. In Sect. 5.3 it is used as a measure of distance between generated and original image. Another method to measure this distance is the mean squared error (**MSE**) which calculates the difference of images based on the squared error between each pixel. The optimum value to be reached between two images is 0.

5.3   Specificity and Generalization Ability

The final model should be able to generate only valid samples of what it has learned from the training images (specificity) and it should be able to represent each of the original images in form of a generated image (generalization ability) [14]. Specificity is calculated by summing up the distance from each sample image to the closest original image and dividing that by the number of generated samples M, as shown in (3). $Y^{(M)} = \{y_a \in \mathbb{R}^n : a = 1,...M\}$ represents the set of generated samples and x_i the original image. The generalization ability is calculated by summing up the distance for each original sample to its closest (most similar) generated image and dividing it by the number of original images as shown in (4), with N being the number of original images. SSIM and MSE are used as distance measures.

$$S(n_m) = \frac{1}{M} \sum_{a=1}^{M} \min_i \|y_a - x_i\| \tag{3}$$

$$G(n_m) = \frac{1}{N} \sum_{i=1}^{N} \min_a \|y_a - x_i\| \qquad (4)$$

6   Evaluation

Our approach is a evaluated qualitatively and quantitatively. The qualitative approach is based on the visual impression. For each dataset, it was possible to generate images that look realistic to a non-expert at first sight. Figure 3 provides samples of the generated images using the hyperparameters specified in Sect. 3. The chosen hyperparameters do not lead to optimal results for each dataset, but show that even with sub-optimal hyperparameters, realistic image synthesis is possible. The quantitative evaluation results can be found in Table 1.

Results generated with the GAN trained on only 115 images outperformed the GAN trained on all chest X-rays when looking at the specificity and generalization ability of the model. The FID score however, is worse for the chest-115 model compared to using all data. Combining these two facts with visual analysis, the worse FID score for the chest-115 model might be due to more blurry images. Worse specificity and generalization ability for the chest-all model may be due to multiple almost completely unrecognizable generated images. Examples for unsuccessful image generations of the two datasets are shown in Fig. 4. In this case, the chest-115 dataset served as the better training set, as more anatomical correctness is represented in the results.

The overall FID values achieved for the generated images correlate to the quality of the visual results. However, the values are still relatively high, compared to some state-of-the-art FID values for natural images [15] that have achieved values as low as 7.4, compared to the lowest value of 77.08 achieved for the non-AMD dataset (see Table 1). This large difference shows that there is still a lot of improvement to be achieved when generating such images.

Observing the specificity and generalization ability of all trained models, the (non-) AMD images achieve better values than the other datasets. This underlines the principle of quality over quantity in the data. Still, quantity should not be neglected as the pneumonia and non-pneumonia images show similar quality, but the better values are achieved by the pneumonia model, as it has almost three-times as many training images.

Principal component analysis (PCA) has been applied to the image data to visualize the original data alongside the generated data in one graph in order to assess the differences of the data and detect outliers (see Fig. 5). The evaluation of PCA component diagrams leads to the conclusion, that although a large group of the generated images blend in with the original images there is still a significant number of outliers. When visually assessing such images, it is obvious why they differ from the other images, as they are usually distorted and do not show a high level of detail. This could most likely be improved by training the model longer or with a different architecture.

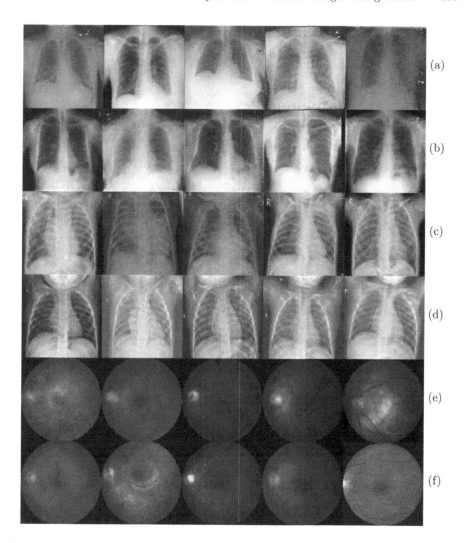

Fig. 3. Examples for generated data using learning rate of 0.0002, batch size 32 and kernel size 5. (a) Chest X-ray using all images, (b) Chest X-ray using dataset of size 115 (c) Pneumonia, (d) Non-pneumonia, (e) AMD, (f) Non-AMD

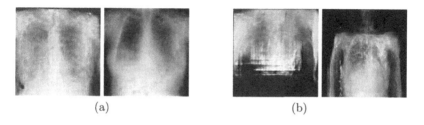

Fig. 4. Examples for bad generated images. (a) Chest-115, (b) Chest-all

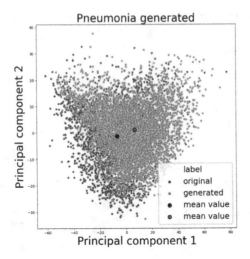

Fig. 5. PCA component diagram of pneumonia data

Table 1. Values for all datasets with a learning rate of 0.0002. Batch size as BS and kernel size as KS. Optimum value is 1 when using SSIM and 0 when using MSE. Best values for each dataset values are printed **bold**.

Dataset	BS	KS	$S(SSIM)$	$G(SSIM)$	$S(MSE)$	$G(MSE)$	FID
AMD	8	3	0.70	0.70	285.71	225.45	102.42
	8	5	0.71	0.72	328.75	211.92	89.33
	32	3	0.72	0.72	190.60	198.13	96.15
	32	5	**0.76**	**0.75**	202.88	182.61	**84.49**
	64	3	0.71	0.71	193.12	186.03	104.03
	64	5	0.74	0.74	**177.63**	**167.07**	89.07
Non-AMD	8	3	0.56	0.53	1049.39	733.22	131.76
	8	5	0.70	0.68	314.87	231.35	**77.08**
	32	3	0.68	0.67	288.05	240.65	84.23
	32	5	0.70	0.69	300.05	239.49	81.21
	64	3	0.69	0.68	**253.40**	220.58	90.71
	64	5	**0.70**	**0.69**	265.64	**206.63**	83.41
Pneumonia	32	3	0.48	0.47	897.96	913.32	121.57
	32	5	**0.50**	**0.48**	**820.72**	**840.02**	128.15
	64	3	0.47	0.46	928.70	930.66	128.31
	64	5	0.50	0.48	869.98	896.65	**119.17**
Non-pneumonia	32	3	0.43	0.41	1092.11	1150.48	135.31
	32	5	**0.45**	**0.43**	1089.70	**1131.42**	131.96
	64	3	0.43	0.41	**1076.56**	1187.16	139.33
	64	5	0.45	0.42	1088.28	1180.62	**130.01**
Chest-all	32	3	0.54	0.52	1113.43	1158.74	163.93
	32	5	0.57	0.54	1191.14	1491.22	162.32
	64	3	0.55	0.53	1206.73	1196.92	160.45
	64	5	**0.58**	**0.55**	**1056.10**	**1131.63**	**157.90**
Chest-115	32	3	0.53	0.52	1328.06	1411.22	272.82
	32	5	**0.66**	**0.63**	**938.32**	**1072.29**	**266.09**
	64	3	0.54	0.52	1312.0	1409.89	296.57
	64	3	0.63	0.6	1005.77	1133.47	295.72

7 Discussion

The presented approach shows that is generally possible to create artificial and realistic looking images from large sets of medical training data. Our assumption is that such methods could be used in the future to alleviate privacy problems and to allow for greater public sharing of data. At the current point in time, however, there are unresolved questions that need to be addressed first. Primarily, legal aspects of data privacy are varying from country to country and often any use of personal information - even if only used implicitly as in the proposed method - requires a consent from the patient. In our view, obtaining such consent could be eased by explaining to the patient that the possibility of reconstructing the original individual data is not possible. One straightforward way could be to only share generated images which have a certain similarity distance to all original images. That way, it would be hard to reconstruct the original images. The question that still remains is, what would be an acceptable visual difference. A possibility could be a manual check by a doctor that focuses on excluding unsuccessful generated images, as well as images that may resemble original data too closely.

Another point of discussion is the medical and anatomical correctness of the generated data. In our view this can only be judged by a medical expert prior to sharing the data. For some use cases such as assessing the anatomical correctness of organ shapes or boundaries, this can be done quite easily by an expert. Training an artificial intelligence algorithm on such artificial and medically approved data should benefit most from the presented concept. Other use cases such as tumours or other pathologies might be more difficult to assess even by an expert and generated artificial images could be too risky to train other algorithms on.

8 Conclusion

The presented approach shows that it is generally possible to generate realistic looking medical images using GANs that do not reveal the patient's personal information. Here, the quality of the training images is of great importance. Implementing such an image generating functionality would require a prepro-cessing step that assures uniformity of the training data as this heavily impacts the generated results. The collected values for the images, such as FID and SSIM can give some guidance, when assessing the accuracy/level of realism of the images, but cannot be used as a standalone method of assessment. Before reaching final conclusions, it is necessary to consult medical specialists to ana-lyze the images regarding anatomical correctness and a match in the diagnosis the images are intended to show. This unsupervised learning method needs to undergo additional training in order to achieve a higher level of realism and min-imize the amount of flawed generated images. The presented approach is seen as a first step towards generating synthetic training data in order to reduce the lack of large medical databases available to the public and therefore to improve data accessibility for researchers and developers to create better and more reliable AI in the medical domain.

References

1. Esteva, A., et al.: Dermatologist-level classification of skin cancer with deep neural networks. Nature **542**, 115–118 (2017)
2. Designed by Freepik
3. iChallenge-AMD. https://amd.grand-challenge.org/. Accessed 15 July 2019
4. Kaggle Chest X-Ray Images (Pneumonia). https://www.kaggle.com/paultimothymooney/chest-xray-pneumonia. Accessed 15 July 2019
5. Goodfellow, I., et al.: Generative adversarial nets. In: Advances in Neural Information Processing Systems (2014)
6. Shin, H.-C., et al.: Medical image synthesis for data augmentation and anonymization using generative adversarial networks. In: Gooya, A., Goksel, O., Oguz, I., Burgos, N. (eds.) SASHIMI 2018. LNCS, vol. 11037, pp. 1–11. Springer, Cham (2018). https://doi.org/10.1007/978-3-030-00536-8_1
7. Korkinof, D., et al.: High-resolution mammogram synthesis using progressive generative adversarial networks (2018)
8. Zhao, H., et al.: Synthesizing retinal and neuronal images with generative adversarial nets. Med. Image Anal. **49**, 14–26 (2018)
9. Gulrajani, I., et al.: Improved training of Wasserstein GANs. CoRR (2017)
10. Arjovski, M., et al.: Wasserstein GAN. ArXiv (2017)
11. Kaggle Random Sample of NIH Chest X-ray Dataset. https://www.kaggle.com/nih-chest-xrays/sample/version/4. Accessed 15 July 2019
12. Heusel, M., et al.: GANs trained by a two time-scale update rule converge to a local Nash equilibrium. In: Advances in Neural Information Processing Systems (2017)
13. Wang, Z., et al.: Image quality assessment: from error visibility to structural similarity. IEEE Trans. Image Process. **13**(4), 600–612 (2004)
14. Davies, R., Twining, C., Taylor, C.: Statistical Models of Shape: Optimisation and Evaluation, pp. 78–79. Springer, Cham (2008). https://doi.org/10.1007/978-1-84800-138-1
15. Brock, A., et al.: Large scale GAN training for high fidelity natural image synthesis. In: International Conference on Learning Representations (2019)

DPANet: A Novel Network Based on Dense Pyramid Feature Extractor and Dual Correlation Analysis Attention Modules for Colon Glands Segmentation

Shuting Liu[1], Baochang Zhang[2], Xi Li[3], Yiqing Liu[1], Mengying Hu[1],
Tian Guan[1(✉)], and Yonghong He[1(✉)]

[1] Graduate School at Shenzhen, Tsinghua University, Beijing, China
{guantian,heyh}@sz.tsinghua.edu.cn
[2] Shenzhen Colleges of Advanced Technology, University of Chinese Academy
of Sciences, Beijing, China
[3] Department of Gastroenterology, Peking University Shenzhen Hospital,
Shenzhen, China

Abstract. Accurate segmentation of glands from histology images is a crucial step to obtain reliable morphological statistics for quantitative diagnosis. However, this task is formidable because of the enormous variability in glandular appearance and the difficulty in distinguishing between glandular and non-glandular histological structures. To address this challenge, a novel neural network is proposed to effectively extract benign or malignant colon glands from histology images. Our network has the following innovations: (1) Under the same resolution space, multi-receptive field pyramid features are captured from dense multi-rate dilated convolution architecture with sounder dilated rate setting for accurate gland segmentation. (2) Furthermore, the extracted features are down-sampled by B-spline algorithm to provide different resolution information for the network. (3) Specifically, we embed spatial-channel soft attention modules before each deconvolution operation in the decoder phase, which can better reintegrate features and support clear semantic similarity for network. All these unique operations boost the performance of our method on gland segmentation task. We achieve state-of-the-art performance on the publicly available Warwick-QU dataset.

Keywords: Colon glands segmentation · Correlation analysis · Attention module · Spatial pyramid feature

1 Introduction

Colorectal cancer is one of the major types of gastrointestinal cancer that threatens the lives of millions of people around the world [1]. Currently, pathological examination has become a common and accurate method in the diagnosis of cancers, such as colon,

This project was supported by grants from the Nature Science Foundation of China (Nos. NSFC81401539 and NSFC31271056) and the projects in the Shenzhen Medical Engineering Laboratory For Human Auditory-equilibrium Function.

© Springer Nature Switzerland AG 2019
H. Greenspan et al. (Eds.): CLIP 2019/UNSURE 2019, LNCS 11840, pp. 135–145, 2019.
https://doi.org/10.1007/978-3-030-32689-0_14

breast and prostate. The digitization of biopsy samples has been an important turning point in the development of pathology, which also promotes the development of pathological statistics. Accurate segmentation of glands from histology images is a crucial step to obtain reliable morphological statistical information for quantitative diagnosis. However, manual annotation suffers from some issues such as poor reproducibility, serious subjective impact and time-consuming. Hence, there is a growing demand for accurate and automatic segmentation method.

Most of the previous methods [2] for gland segmentation are model-driven methods which roughly be divided into three classes: (i) threshold methods based on color intensities, (ii) graphic model methods, (iii) hybrid methods based on the multi-level information in the histology image. Nevertheless, these methods usually cannot make a satisfying segmentation result of malignant glandular histology image. Later, the data-driven approach attracts the attention of many researchers. Xu et al. [3] employed a convolutional neural network (CNN) based on sliding window strategy for a supervised pixel classification to automatically segment or classify epithelial and stromal regions from digitized tumor tissue micro-arrays, which greatly outperformed the hand-crafted feature-based methods. However, the sliding window strategy is time-consuming.

U-Net [4] as an end-to-end network has successfully overcome the time-consuming problem and achieved excellent performance in the task of cell segmentation. To further improve the segmentation performance, Chen et al. [5] proposed a deep contour aware network (DCAN) to segment the gland body and contour respectively, and achieved the best performance in the challenge of MICCAI gland segmentation (GlaS) [6] in 2015. Xu et al. [7] built a framework that automatically exploits and fuses complex multi-channel information, regional and boundary patterns, with deep supervision on side responses in gland histology images. Then they improve performance by adding additional object box information. Recently, Raza et al. [8] proposed a multi-input and multi-output network (MIMO-Net), which achieved the new state-of-the-art performance on the publicly available Warwick-QU dataset [6].

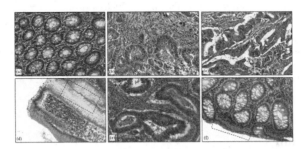

Fig. 1. Some samples of colon glands histology image. (a) benign; (b, c) malignant; (d) sticky glands; (e) artifacts (f) inconsistencies appearance. In subfigures (a, b): Lumen (black line), cytoplasm (green line), epithelial cells (blue line), and stroma (red line). (Color figure online)

However, the accurate and automatic segmentation of colon glands is still a challenge issue, the main reasons are summarized as follows: (1) due to the differentiations of histologic grades, there is a huge variety in shape, size, and texture of glands (2) typically, a colon gland contains four tissue components: lumen, cytoplasm, epithelial cells, and stroma. However, the glandular structures have seriously degenerated in malignant cases. (3) the existence of sticky glands in histology image makes it quite hard for automated methods to separate objects individually. (4) staining also cause deformation, artifacts and inconsistencies in the appearance of the tissue, which hinder the segmentation process. Figure 1 shows the great differences in glandular structure.

In this paper, we proposed a dual pyramid attention network (DPANet) to segment benign or malignant colon glands from histology images. The base-bone network in our method is an encoder-decoder U-shape network which can fuse the mid-level and high-level semantic features to obtain different scale context. In order to further improve the performance of base-bone network, the improvements between the proposed model with respect to base-bone network are threefold. Firstly, we embed the dense multi-rate dilated convolution (DMDC) unit into the feature extraction encoder part, which consists of multi-rates dilated convolution operations with a dense connection. Hence, dense pyramid features with different receptive fields are extracted. Secondly, we adopt B-spline algorithm to down-sample the features extracted from the previous layer and took them as a part of input of the current layer, which provides different resolution feature information for the network with the minimal information loss. Thirdly, in the decoder phase, a dual pyramid attention (DPA) architecture is proposed, which connects the DMDC units with the spatial-channel attention modules to capture global contextual information in the spatial and channel dimensions. In addition, we design a weight map for the loss function and perform high-weight-supervised training on the gland contour. Our approach has been confirmed the effectiveness through extensive experiments on the benchmark dataset of gland segmentation (GlaS) challenge contest in MICCAI 2015, which has better performance than other methods.

2   Dual Pyramid Attention Network

An overview of the proposed dual pyramid attention network is shown in Fig. 2, which consist of encoder and decoder.

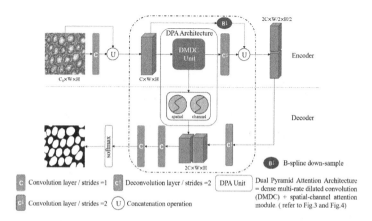

Fig. 2. An overview of dual pyramid attention network. (Note: the architecture in the black dotted box is four-fold in the whole network)

The encoder starts with a convolution with kernel size of 3×3 and stride of 1 on $512 \times 512 \times 3$ input images. The channel concatenation is then performed between the original input image and first extracted feature maps, which helps the original image information spread all over the encoder phase. The following part architecture that located in the black dotted box in the Fig. 2. is the key step of the whole DPANet, which mainly consists of DMDC unit (as shown in Fig. 3) of the encoder part and spatial-channel attention modules (as shown in Fig. 4) of decoder part. In order to maintain the spatial continuity of features, there does not exist any pooling operation, which is instead by the convolution with a stride of 2 or B-spline down-sampling. It is worth the note that each convolution layer (shown by purple box in Fig. 2) is a series of operations, i.e. convolution with a kernel of size 3×3, batch normalization, activation layer (such as ReLU) and dropout operation. In addition, aims to recover the resolution of the feature map from 32×32 to 512×512, deconvolution is adopted to up-sample the feature map. Finally, we obtain the final segmentation mask by a 1×1 convolution and a softmax activation function.

The proposed DPANet consists of three major components: (I) The DMDC units used for pyramid feature extraction. (II) The spatial-channel attention modules highlight salient features extracted by DMDC unit. (III) The designed loss function is utilized for addressing the problem of foreground-background class imbalance and the existence of sticky glands.

2.1   Dense Multi-rate Dilated Convolution Unit (DMDC)

Dilated convolution expand feature reception field without sacrificing feature spatial resolution. Deeplabv3 [9] embedded atrous spatial pyramid pooling (ASPP) unit on the top of decoder to exploit multi-scale contextual information, which consists of parallel dilated convolution with different rates. Then, Yang et al. [10] employed cascading and parallel strategies on dilated convolution and then pushed a novel architecture which generated much more densely scaled receptive fields than [9]. The variants of dilated convolution have shown superior performance on scene object recognition task. In this work, we not only embed DMDC unit (as shown in Fig. 2) on the top of decoder part as same as [9, 10], but also combine it with each feature extraction layer of U-shape. Thereby multi-scale contextual information is obtained at different spatial resolutions.

However, the computation nodes of dilated convolution with different dilated rate are similar to sparse grids, which are some independent sets from the previous layers. Dilated convolution obtains a larger feature reception field, but the local information is lost, which make the long-range information lack correlation, especially the case of the dilated rate being bigger than the object's radium. The previous variants of dilated convolution such as ASPP are beneficial to capture the large gland objects, whereas they are not good for small objects. DenseASPP proposed by Yang et $al.$ [10] is constructed with dilation rates of 3, 6, 12, 18. The dense connection strategy potentially includes the cascade structure of dilated convolution, which alleviates the loss of local contextual information to some extent. However, their dilated rates are still too sparse to fully utilize all the information under the specific reception field.

In order to obtain multi-scale information without losing local information, we further explore the setting of the dilated rate of the cascading dilated convolutions. In the Nth layer We assume the 1-dimension dilated convolutional with dilation rate of R_d^n and a kernel size of K_d^n, the equivalent receptive field (RF) size is:

$$RF = \left(R_d^n - 1\right) \times \left(K_d^n - 1\right) + K_d^n \tag{1}$$

However, $\left(R_d^n - 1\right) \times \left(K_d^n - 1\right)$ nodes are not involved in the calculation. As a transition, in the former layer, we assume that a traditional 1-dimension convolution is needed, and the kernel size of K^{n-1} is

$$K^{n-1} = \left\lceil \left(R_d^n - 1\right)/2 \right\rceil \times 2 + 1 \tag{2}$$

Therefore, in the $N - 1^{th}$ layer, the dilated rate R_d^{n-1} of the cascading dilated convolution with a manual settings kernel size of K_d^{n-1} should not bigger than the upper limit $sup\left(R_d^{n-1}\right)$ which is defined as follow:

$$sup\left(R_d^{n-1}\right) = \left\lceil \left\lceil \left(K^{n-1} - K_d^{n-1}\right)/\left(K_d^{n-1} + 1\right)\right\rceil/2 \right\rceil \times 2 + 1 \tag{3}$$

We continue to derive backward according to formula (1–3) until $sup\left(R_d^i\right) = 1$. Figure 3(a) shows the architecture of DMDC unit, where three 3×3 dilated convolutions with dilation rate of 1, 2, 3 and a 1×1 tradition convolution are employed to capture multi-scale denser pyramid features with minimum local contextual information loss. According to formula (1–3), the setting of dilation rates is very sound. Then, we concatenate the features and then a 1×1 tradition convolution is used to recognize the feature maps. Figure 3(b) illustrates scale pyramid corresponding to the setting of densely dilated convolutions with dilation rates of 1, 2, 3, while the size of corresponding reception filed.

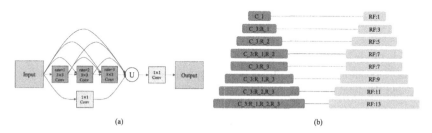

(a)   (b)

Fig. 3. (a) The architecture of DMDC unit and (b) the scale pyramid corresponding to the dilation rates of 1, 2, 3.

2.2   Spatial-Channel Attention Module

Many works [11] suggest that only using local context information may lead to misclassification of objects, which means that only relying on more local features cannot get more accurate gland segmentation. In order to make the network know more global information, we propose a spatial-channel attention module as shown in Fig. 4, which better reintegrate features and support clear semantic similarity for network.

As illustrated in Fig. 4, given a local dense pyramid feature A obtained by DMDC unit, we feed it into spatial attention module and channel attention module respectively. The two-path attention module implements similar operations. The main difference is that spatial attention module focuses on the correlation between any two spatial positions in feature map, while channel attention module focuses on the correlation between any two channels. we take the spatial attention module as an example of a detailed description.

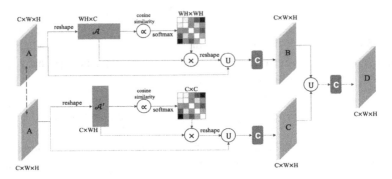

Fig. 4. The structure of spatial-channel attention module. Spatial attention module (up) and channel attention module (down)

We firstly reshape the feature map $A \in R^{C \times W \times H}$ to the matrix $\mathcal{A}$ with shape of $WH \times C$. Then, we use cosine similarity to compute the correlation $Coor_{i,j}$ between any two positions:

$$Coor_{i,j} = \frac{f_i \cdot f_i}{\|f\|_i \cdot \|f_j\|}. \tag{4}$$

where f_i is the feature vector in i^{th} position of the feature map A and f_j is the feature vector in j^{th} position. Then a softmax activation function is employed to normalize the $Coor_{i,j}$ and the final attention matrix S is obtained:

$$S_{i,j} = \frac{\exp(Coor_{i,j})}{\sum_{j=1}^{WH} \exp(Coor_{i,j})} \tag{5}$$

where $S_{i,j}$ measure the impact of the i_{th} position on the j_{th} position. Then we perform a matrix multiplication between the spatial attention matrix S and the feature matrix $\mathcal{A}$ and reshape the result to $R^{C \times W \times H}$. Finally, we concatenate the result with input feature map A and use a 1×1 convolution to reintegrate the features. Therefore, both the local contextual information and global similarity information are cleverly combined, which maintain the semantic consistency and improve the network performance.

2.3   Loss Function

In the task of gland segmentation, because of the imbalance ratio between the foreground and the background in each histology images, we firstly employ the balanced weight dice loss to address this problem. Secondly, due to both benign to malignant glands having significant contour characteristic, we design a contour weight map to perform high-weighted supervised training on the gland contour region as shown in Fig. 5. Moreover, we add the L2 regularization term into the loss function to prevent overfitting. Therefore, the final loss function $\mathcal{L}(x, \vartheta)$ is defined as follows:

$$
\begin{cases}
\mathcal{L}(x, \vartheta) = \mathcal{L}_b(p(x), g(x), w_b, w_c) + \mathcal{L}_c(p(x), g(x), w_c) + \lambda \|\vartheta\|^2 \\
\mathcal{L}_b(p(x), g(x), w_b, w_c) = 1 - \sum_{k=1}^{N=2} \frac{2*\sum_i w_b*(w_c+1)*p_{k,i}*g_{k,i}}{\sum_i w_b*(w_c+1)*(p_{k,i}+g_{k,i})} \\
\mathcal{L}_c(p(x), g(x), w_c) = 1 - \sum_{k=1}^{N=2} \frac{2*\sum_i w_{c,k}*p_{k,i}*g_{k,i}}{\sum_i w_{c,k}*(p_{k,i}+g_{k,i})}
\end{cases}
\tag{6}
$$

where ϑ is the trainable parameters in the network. $p(x)$ is the hotmap outputted by the network and $g(x)$ is the one-hot map of ground truth. The balance weight map $w_b = \{1/\sum_i g_{k,i}, i = 1, 2\}$ and the contour weight map w_c is computed by the follows equations:

$$
\begin{cases}
d_{i,j} = \min\{dist(\widetilde{g}_b, i, j) \cup dist(g_o[k], i, j) | k = 1 \cdots n\} \\
w_{c\,i,j}^0(d_{i,j}, w_0, \sigma) = w_0 exp\left(-d_{i,j}^2/(2\sigma^2)\right) \\
w_{c\,i,j} = \begin{cases} 0 & if\ w_{c\,i,j}^0 < w_c^0(r, w_0, \sigma) \\ w_{c\,i,j}^0 & if\ w_{c\,i,j}^0 > w_c^0(r, w_0, \sigma) \end{cases}
\end{cases}
\tag{7}
$$

where $dist(*)$ is used to calculate the distance between each non-zero point in the image and its nearest zero point. $\widetilde{g}_b$ is the label-map where background is 1 and gland objects is $0.g_o[k]$ is the label-map where only the kth gland object is 1. In this work, we set w_0 to 1.0, σ to 15 and r to 15. The balance weight map and the contour weight map is shown in Fig. 5.

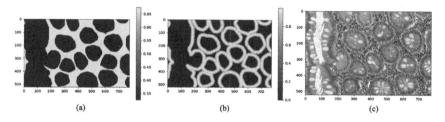

(a)   (b)   (c)

Fig. 5. (a) The balance weight map, (b) the contour weight map generated by Eq. (7) and (c) the corresponding image

3 Experiment and Result

3.1 Dataset and Data Augmentation

We evaluated our method on the public dataset of Gland Segmentation (GlaS) Challenge Contest in MICCAI 2015. The images were acquired by a Zeiss MIRAX MIDI slide scanner from colorectal cancer tissues with a resolution of 0.62 μm/pixel. These 165 images, including a wide range histological grades from benign to malignant subjects, consisted of 85 training images (37 benign and 48 malignant) and 80 testing images (37 benign and 43 malignant). Furthermore, the testing images are split into two test sets: Test A (60 images) and Test B (20 images).

To increase the robustness and reduce overfitting, we utilized the strategy of data augmentation to enlarge the dataset. Our augmentations include flip, rotation, random crop, Gaussian noise, elastic transform, brightness transform, color jittering.

3.2 Implementation Details

Before feeding the data to the network, we normalize the data with the mean of 0 and standard deviation of 1. All the parameters in the convolutional layers are initialized according to He *et al.*'s work [12]. We set the λ in L2 regularization to 0.0001 and utilize stochastic gradient descent to minimize the loss, meanwhile, the learning rate was set as 0.0005 initially and decreased using exponential decay with the decay rate of 0.9 and the decay step of 2000. The batch size is 8. The network is trained on a computer with Intel Core i7-6850 k CPU, 128 GB RAM, and three NVidia GTX 1080-Ti GPUs.

Then, post-processing steps including filling holes and removing small areas are performed on the segmentation results using. Finally, each connected component is labeled with a unique value for representing one segmented gland.

3.3 Quantification Result

The performance of the proposed DPANet is evaluated by using the same evaluation criteria used in the MICCAI 2015 GlaS challenge [8], consisting of F1 score $(F1_{score})$, object-level Dice $(Dice_{obj})$ and object-level Hausdorff distance (H_{obj}). The F1 score is employed to measure the detection accuracy of individual glandular objects, the object-level Dice is a measure of similarity between two sets of samples and the Hausdorff distance measures the boundary-based segmentation accuracy.

As can be seen from Table 1, our proposed network achieves the advanced performance compared to the methods in the 2015 MICCAI GlaS Challenge dataset. Our proposed method gets higher scores at the metrics of object-level Dice and object-level Hausdorff distance than all the other methods. Especially, we make a great improvement on test-B dataset, which makes a 5.2% increment on the object-level Dice and reduces the Hausdorff distance by about 45.51. Overall, our proposed DPANnet rank the top one. Figure 6 further represents our segmentation results is more accurate and sensitive to the gland contour. Compared our result with that of U-net, there are many misclassification regions in the result of U-net, which suggests that our method capture

Table 1. Comparative analysis of models on the GlaS challenge dataset.

Methods	$F1_{score}$				$Dice_{obj}$				H_{obj}				$R\_$ Sum
	Test A		Test B		Test A		Test B		Test A		Test B		
	S	R	S	R	S	R	S	R	S	R	S	R	
Our DPANet	0.892	4	**0.773**	1	0.902	2	**0.852**	1	**43.91**	1	**102.07**	1	*10*
MIMONet [7]	**0.913**	1	0.724	4	**0.906**	1	0.785	6	49.15	3	133.98	3	*18*
Xu et al. [8]	0.858	9	0.771	2	0.888	4	0.815	2	54.20	4	129.93	2	*23*
CUmed2: DCAN	0.912	2	0.716	6	0.897	3	0.781	8	45.42	2	160.35	9	*30*
ExB1	0.891	6	0.703	7	0.882	7	0.786	4	57.41	9	145.58	4	*37*
ExB3	0.896	3	0.719	5	0.886	5	0.765	9	57.36	8	159.87	8	*38*
Freib2:Unet	0.870	7	0.695	8	0.876	8	0.786	5	57.09	6	148.47	6	*40*
CUmed1: DCAN	0.868	8	0.769	3	0.867	10	0.800	3	74.6	10	153.65	7	*41*
ExB2	0.892	4	0.686	9	0.884	6	0.754	10	54.79	5	187.44	11	*45*
Freib1:Unet	0.834	10	0.605	10	0.875	9	0.783	7	57.19	7	146.61	5	*48*
CVML	0.652	12	0.541	11	0.644	13	0.654	11	155.43	13	176.24	10	*70*
LIB	0.777	11	0.306	13	0.781	11	0.617	12	112.71	12	190.45	12	*71*
vision4Glas	0.635	13	0.527	12	0.737	12	0.610	13	107.49	11	210.10	13	*74*

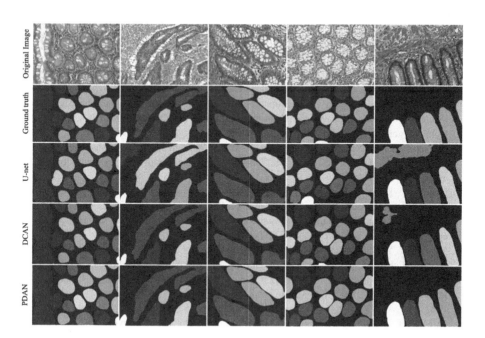

Fig. 6. The gland segmentation results of different methods on the GlaS dataset.

more effective features and only utilizing the local contextual information is not sufficient to lead an accurate segment. Meanwhile, the previous top one method DCAN proposed by Chen *et al.* [5] made an additional segmentation on the gland contour and then fused the segmentation result, which leads the gland contour in final segmentation was usually smaller than that in ground truth. Comparing with DCAN, our method obtain superior gland segmentation and describe the edge more accurately.

4 Conclusion

In this paper, we presented a deep dual pyramid attention network to accurately segment glands from histology images. The proposed network employed B-spline downsampling to retain maximal pre-learned information during feature extraction, which is very important for successful gland instance segmentation. In order to self-adapt glands of various sizes, we use DMDC unit with sounder dilated rate setting for effective multi-scale aggregation. Furthermore, spatial and channel attention modules are explored to support global contextual information and semantic feature consistency. Extensive experimental results on the benchmark dataset proved the good performance of the proposed method. In future work, we will optimize the method and investigate its capability on large-scale histopathological datasets.

References

1. Moridikia, A.: Potential candidates for diagnosis and treatment of colorectal cancer. J. Cell. Physiol. **233**(2), 901–913 (2018)
2. Kainz, P.: Segmentation and classification of colon glands with deep convolutional neural networks and total variation regularization. PeerJ **5**, e3874 (2017)
3. Xu, Y.: Large scale tissue histopathology image classification, segmentation, and visualization via deep convolutional activation features. BMC Bioinform. **18**(1), 281 (2017)
4. Ronneberger, O., Fischer, P., Brox, T.: U-Net: convolutional networks for biomedical image segmentation. In: Navab, N., Hornegger, J., Wells, William M., Frangi, Alejandro F. (eds.) MICCAI 2015. LNCS, vol. 9351, pp. 234–241. Springer, Cham (2015). https://doi.org/10.1007/978-3-319-24574-4_28
5. Chen, H.: DCAN: deep contour-aware networks for accurate gland segmentation. In: The IEEE conference on Computer Vision and Pattern Recognition, pp. 2487–2496 (2016)
6. Sirinukunwattana, K.: Gland segmentation in colon histology images: the glas challenge contest. Med. Image Anal. **35**, 489–502 (2017)
7. Xu, Y., Li, Y., Liu, M., Wang, Y., Lai, M., Chang, E.I.-C.: Gland instance segmentation by deep multichannel side supervision. In: Ourselin, S., Joskowicz, L., Sabuncu, Mert R., Unal, G., Wells, W. (eds.) MICCAI 2016. LNCS, vol. 9901, pp. 496–504. Springer, Cham (2016). https://doi.org/10.1007/978-3-319-46723-8_57
8. Raza, S.E.A., Cheung, L., Epstein, D., Pelengaris, S., Khan, M., Rajpoot, Nasir M.: MIMONet: gland segmentation using multi-input-multi-output convolutional neural network. In: Valdés Hernández, M., González-Castro, V. (eds.) MIUA 2017. CCIS, vol. 723, pp. 698–706. Springer, Cham (2017). https://doi.org/10.1007/978-3-319-60964-5_61

9. Chen, L.C.: Deeplab: semantic image segmentation with deep convolutional nets, atrous convolution, and fully connected crfs. IEEE Trans. Pattern Anal. Mach. Intell. **40**(4), 834–848 (2017)

10. Yang, M.: DenseASPP for semantic segmentation in street scenes. In: Proceedings of the IEEE Conference on Computer Vision and Pattern Recognition, pp. 3684–3692 (2016)

11. Zhao, H., Zhang, Y., Liu, S., Shi, J., Loy, C.C., Lin, D., Jia, J.: PSANet: point-wise spatial attention network for scene parsing. In: Ferrari, V., Hebert, M., Sminchisescu, C., Weiss, Y. (eds.) ECCV 2018. LNCS, vol. 11213, pp. 270–286. Springer, Cham (2018). https://doi.org/10.1007/978-3-030-01240-3_17

12. He, K.: Delving deep into rectifiers: surpassing human-level performance on imagenet classification. In: The IEEE International Conference on Computer Vision, pp. 1026–1034 (2015)

Multi-instance Deep Learning with Graph Convolutional Neural Networks for Diagnosis of Kidney Diseases Using Ultrasound Imaging

Shi Yin[1,2]([envelope]), Qinmu Peng[1], Hongming Li[2], Zhengqiang Zhang[1], Xinge You[1], Hangfan Liu[2], Katherine Fischer[5,6], Susan L. Furth[4], Gregory E. Tasian[3,5,6], and Yong Fan[2]

[1] School of Electronic Information and Communications, Huazhong University of Science and Technology, Wuhan, China
yinshi.wh@gmail.com
[2] Department of Radiology, Perelman School of Medicine, University of Pennsylvania, Philadelphia, PA 19104, USA
[3] Department of Biostatistics, Epidemiology, and Informatics, University of Pennsylvania, Philadelphia, PA 19104, USA
[4] Department of Pediatrics, The Children's Hospital of Philadelphia, Philadelphia, PA 19104, USA
[5] Department of Surgery, Division of Pediatric Nephrology, The Children's Hospital of Philadelphia, Philadelphia, PA 19104, USA
[6] Center for Pediatric Clinical Effectiveness, The Children's Hospital of Philadelphia, Philadelphia, PA 19104, USA

Abstract. Ultrasound imaging (US) is commonly used in nephrology for diagnostic studies of the kidneys and lower urinary tract. However, it remains challenging to automate the disease diagnosis based on clinical 2D US images since they provide partial anatomic information of the kidney and the 2D images of the same kidney may have heterogeneous appearance. To overcome this challenge, we develop a novel multi-instance deep learning method to build a robust classifier by treating multiple 2D US images of each individual subject as multiple instances of one bag. Particularly, we adopt convolutional neural networks (CNNs) to learn instance-level features from 2D US kidney images and graph convolutional networks (GCNs) to further optimize the instance-level features by exploring potential correlation among instances of the same bag. We also adopt a gated attention-based MIL pooling to learn bag-level features using full-connected neural networks (FCNs). Finally, we integrate both instance-level and bag-level supervision to further improve the bag-level classification accuracy. Ablation studies and comparison results have demonstrated that our method could accurately diagnose kidney diseases using ultrasound imaging, with better performance than alternative state-of-the-art multi-instance deep learning methods.

Keywords: Automatic diagnosis · Ultrasound imaging · Graph convolutional neural networks · Multi-instance learning

© Springer Nature Switzerland AG 2019
H. Greenspan et al. (Eds.): CLIP 2019/UNSURE 2019, LNCS 11840, pp. 146–154, 2019.
https://doi.org/10.1007/978-3-030-32689-0_15

1 Introduction

Ultrasound imaging (US) is commonly used in nephrology for diagnostic studies of the kidneys and urinary tract. Anatomic measures of the kidney computed from US data, such as renal parenchymal area, are correlated with kidney function [1], and pattern classifiers built upon US imaging features could aid kidney disease diagnosis [2, 3]. Recent deep learning studies have demonstrated that automated US data analysis could achieve promising performance in a variety of US data analysis tasks, including segmentation and classification [4–6]. However, it remains challenging to automate the kidney disease diagnosis based on clinical 2D US scans since in clinical practice multiple 2D US scans of the same kidney in different views are often collected and the multi-view 2D US scans have heterogeneous appearance, providing partial anatomic information of the kidney, as illustrated by Fig. 1. Therefore, it is desired to develop a clinically useful diagnosis model that is robust to different views of US images of the same kidney.

Multiple instance learning (MIL) is an ideal tool to build a robust classifier on multi-view 2D US scans of the same kidneys by treating multi-views of 2D US scans of the same kidney as multiple instances of a bag and predicting a bag-level classification label [7]. To effectively solve the MIL classification problem, a number of methods have been developed [7]. Among the existing MIL methods, neural network based methods have demonstrated promising performance in a variety of MIL problems, partially due to its end-to-end learning capability [8–11]. Particularly, neural networks could be used to estimate instance-level classification probabilities and fuse them with a log-sum-exp based max operator [8] or a max operator [9] to generate a bag-level classification probability in an end-to-end learning framework. Since the instance-level classification might be affected by instance label instability problem [12], several embedded-space based deep MIL methods have been developed to learn informative features at the instance level, generate a bag mapping with a permutation-invariant MIL pooling operator, and build a bag-level classifier on the embedded-space in an end-to-end learning framework [10, 11]. Particularly, an attention-based MIL pooling has been develop to learn a weighted average of instances [11].

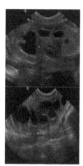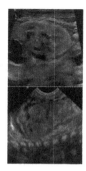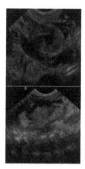

Fig. 1. Multi-view 2D US scans of the same kidney. The images shown on the 1st column have abnormal appearance annotated by radiologists, while others shown on the 2nd and 3rd columns have heterogeneous appearance.

However, the existing deep MIL methods ignore classification labels of instances that are often available in training data and could potentially improve the MIL classification performance if properly integrated, such as those shown on the 1st column of Fig. 1. Furthermore, potential correlation between instances of the same bag has not been well explored in the existing deep MIL methods, which may lead to suboptimal instance-level features. In order to overcome these limitations and further improve deep MIL methods, we develop a novel deep MIL method to learn a deep MIL classification model in an end-to-end learning framework, and apply it to kidney disease diagnosis based on multi-view 2D US images. Particularly, we build a MIL classifier to distinguish kidneys from patients with different kidney diseases based on their multi-view 2D US images. We adopt convolutional neural networks (CNNs) [13] to learn informative US image features, and adopt graph convolutional neural networks (GCNs) [14] as a permutation-invariant operator to further optimize the instance-level CNN features by exploring potential correlation among different instances of the same bag. We adopt the attention-based MIL pooling to learn an optimal permutation-invariant MIL pooling operator in conjunction with learning a bag-level classifier on the embedded space [11]. We further adopt instance-level supervision to enhance the learning of instance features with a focus on instances with reliable labels in the training data. We have validated our method based on clinical 2D US images collected from patients at a local hospital. Extensive comparison and ablation studies have demonstrated that the proposed method could improve the deep MIL methods.

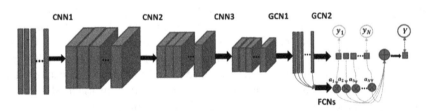

Fig. 2. Network architecture of the proposed deep MIL method. The instance-level supervision is denoted by the yellow circles and the bag-level supervision is denoted by the red circle. (Color figure online)

2   Methodology

We model the kidney disease diagnosis problem based on multi-view 2D US kidney images as a MIL classification problem. Particularly, given kidneys $X_i, i = 1, \ldots, N$, and their 2D US scans in different views, $x_{ik}, k = 1, \ldots, K$, their class label $Y_i = 0$ if all x_{ik} are normal, otherwise $Y_i = 1$. We build a deep MIL network upon recent advances in deep MIL methods that facilitate end-to-end optimization of learning informative features at the instance level, generate a bag mapping with a permutation-invariant MIL pooling operator to embed bags into an embedded-space, and build a bag-level classifier on the embedded-space [10, 11]. As illustrated by Fig. 2, our network consists of CNNs to learn instance-level features from 2D US kidney images, GCNs as permutation-invariant operators to further improve instance-level features, the attention-based MIL pooling to learn a bag-level classifier using full connected neural networks (FCNs), and instance-level supervision to enhance the instance level feature learning and the bag-level classification.

2.1 Learning Image Features for Instances Using CNNs and GCNs with Instance-Level Supervision

To learn informative image features from 2D US kidney images, we adopt CNNs in conjunction with nonlinear activation functions, as illustrated by Fig. 2. Particularly, each 2D US kidney image, x_{ik}, is first fed into multiple layers of CNNs followed by nonlinear activation functions (in the present study, we use 3 CNN layers and *ReLU* activation). We denote the CNN output of x_{ik} by h_{ik}.

As illustrated by Fig. 1, instances of the same bag are potentially correlated with each other. Such correlation information could not be utilized by the CNNs since they are applied to individual instances of the same bag separately. For modeling such unorganized instances, graph theory-based modeling provides an effective means. By modeling each instance as a graph node, and connecting every pair of instances weighted by their similarity measure, we could model the instances with an undirected graph in a graph convolutional network (GCN) framework [14]. Particularly, new features on the graph nodes could be learned by optimizing weights of GCNs.

Given the CNN features of different instances of the same bag, $h_{ik}, k = 1, \ldots, K$, we build a bag-level graph $G = \{V, E\}$ by treating each instance as a graph node and connecting each pair of nodes with a weight measuring their similarity based on their CNN features. GCNs are then adopted to learn new features on the graph nodes [14]:

$$H^{(l+1)} = \sigma(\tilde{D}^{-\frac{1}{2}} A \tilde{D}^{-\frac{1}{2}} (H^{(l)})^T W^{(l)}), \tag{1}$$

where A with its element denoted by a_{ij} is a symmetric adjacent matrix of the undirected graph G, $\tilde{D}_{ii} = \sum_j a_{ij}$ is its degree matrix, $W^{(l)}$ is a layer-specific trainable weight matrix of GCNs, $\sigma(\cdot)$ is a nonlinear activation function, $H_i^{(l)} = \{h_{i1}^l, h_{i2}^l, \ldots, h_{iK}^l\}, h_{ik}^l \in R^F$ is a set of node features obtained by the lth GCN layer, $H_i^{(l+1)} = \{h_{i1}^{l+1}, h_{i2}^{l+1}, \ldots, h_{iK}^{l+1}\}, h_k^{l+1} \in R^M$ is a set of new nodal features obtained by the $(l+1)^{th}$ GCN layer, K is the number of nodes, F and M are the numbers of features on each node obtained by the lth and the $(l+1)^{th}$ GCN layers, respectively.

In the present study, we adopt a Euclidean distance function to obtain the adjacency matrix based on the input feature $H^{(l)}$:

$$a_{ij} = exp\left(-\left\|h_i^l - h_j^l\right\|^2\right). \tag{2}$$

To guide the feature learning, an instance-level supervision is adopted. Particularly, instances with reliable positive labels and all negative instances are used to optimize the feature learning using a softmax loss function. For a two-layer GCN, its forward model takes the simple form:

$$Z = f(H^l) = A_2\text{ReLU}\left(A_1(H^{(0)})^T W^0\right)W^1, \tag{3}$$

where $W^{(0)} \in R^{F \times M}$ and $W^{(l)} \in R^{M \times 2}$ are GCN weight matrices, $H^{(0)}$ is the input CNN features, $A_{i=1,2}$ is the ith layer adjacency matrix which is computed based on the ith layer input features. The second GCN layer yields the instance-level feature $Z^T = \{z_1, z_2, \ldots, z_K\}$ with $z_k \in R^2$, and the instance-level classification probability $P^T = \{p_1, p_2, \ldots, p_K\}$ is obtained by applying a row-wise softmax activation function.

2.2   Attention-Based MIL Pooling Layer with a Gating Mechanism

Once we obtain the instance-level features, we aggregate them to obtain an embedded-space representation using a MIL pooling operator. Instead of adopting simple mean or max MIL pooling, we adopt a gated attention-based MIL pooling layer [11]. Particularly, the attention-based MIL pooling layer learns a weighted average operator to aggregate instance features with a gating mechanism. Given a bag of K instances with GCN features $H^{l+1} = \{h_1^{l+1}, h_2^{l+1}, \ldots, h_K^{l+1}\}, h_k^{l+1} \in R^M$, gated attention-based MIL pooling weight a_k is computed as

$$a_k = \frac{\exp\{w^T\left(\tanh\left(V(h_k^{l+1})^T\right) \bullet \text{sigm}\left(U(h_k^{l+1})^T\right)\right)}{\sum_{j=1}^K \exp\left\{w^T\left(\tanh\left(V(h_j^{l+1})^T\right) \bullet \text{sigm}\left(U(h_j^{l+1})^T\right)\right)\right\}}, \tag{4}$$

where $w \in R^{L \times 1}$ and $V, U \in R^{L \times M}$ are parameters to be optimized, $\bullet$ is an element-wise multiplication, sigm $(\cdot)$ is the sigmoid non-linear activation function, and tanh $(\cdot)$ is used as the gating mechanism. So, the embedded-space representation of bag Z_X is defined as:

$$Z_X = \sum_{k=1}^K a_k z_k. \tag{5}$$

Once the embedded-space representation of bags is obtained, a softmax operation is applied to obtain the bag positive score P_X.

2.3   Jointly Training the Instance-Level and Bag-Level Loss Functions

Once the bag positive score P_X is obtained, the bag-level loss function is defined as:

$$L_X = -\{YlnP_X + (1 - Y)\ln(1 - P_X)\}, \tag{6}$$

To utilize information of instances with reliable labels, we also generate instance-level classification results by optimizing a cross-entropy loss function.

$$L_M = -\sum_{n \in N_Y} \sum_{c=1}^2 y_{nc}lnp_{nc}, \tag{7}$$

where p_{nc} is the classification probability of an instance, y_{nc} is its ground truth classification label, and N_Y is the set of node indices that have reliable classification labels in a bag X. Finally, an overall loss function is defined as:

$$L = L_M + L_X. \tag{8}$$

3   Experimental Results

3.1   Clinical US Kidney Scans

We evaluated our method based on a data set of clinical US kidney scans of kidney patients collected at the Children's Hospital of Philadelphia (CHOP). The work described has been carried out in accordance with the Declaration of Helsinki. The study has been reviewed and approved by the institutional review board.

Participants were randomly sampled from two patient groups. Particularly, one group of the patients were children with mild hydronephrosis (MH) which does not affect the echogenicity, growth, or function of the affected or contralateral normal kidney. The other group of the patients were children with Congenital anomalies of the kidneys and urinary tract (CAKUT), with varying degrees of increased cortical echogenicity, decreased corticomedullary differentiation, and hydronephrosis. All images were obtained for routine clinical care. The first US scans after birth were used, and all identifying information was removed. In total, we obtained 105 MH patients with 2246 scans and 120 CAKUT patients with 2687 scans. All the MH scans were labeled as negative instances with reliable classification labels, all CAKUT scans were labeled as positive instances, and 335 of CAKUT scans with noticeable abnormality from different patients were deemed as instances with reliable classification labels. All the US scans were resized to have a spatial resolution of 321×321, and their image intensities were linearly scaled to [0, 255].

3.2   Implementation Details

Our network consisted of 3 layers of CNNs, and their numbers of channels were set to 128, 64 and 32 respectively. All the CNNs had the same kernel sizes of 5×5 and the same stride sizes of 2. Our GCNs had 2 layers, and their numbers of hidden features were set to 64. In the attention-based MIL pooling network, the number of hidden

Table 1. Comparison results of different versions of the proposed method (mean±std).

Method	Accuracy (mean±std)
Bag-level MILNN	0.852 ± 0.058
Bag-level MILNN+attention	0.852 ± 0.016
Bag-level MILNN+GNN+attention	0.869 ± 0.000
Bag-level MILNN+GNN+attention+all instance supervised	0.869 ± 0.064
Proposed	0.886 ± 0.032

nodes L was set to 64. The learning rate was 0.0001 and batch size was set as 6. The maximum number of iteration steps was set to 20000. All the methods were implemented using TensorFlow and executed on a GeForce GTX 6.00 GB GPU.

3.3 Ablation Studies and Comparisons with Alternative Methods

We compared the proposed network with its degraded versions to investigate how GCNs, the attention-based MIL pooling, and the instance-level supervision contribute to the overall classification based on validation datasets. All the networks had the same number of parameters. Particularly, we first implemented the proposed network with only the bag-level loss function (Bag-level MINN), but without the GCNs (replaced the GCNs with FCNs having the same hidden nodes), the attention-based MIL pooling, and the instance-level loss. Then, Bag-level MINN was enhanced by adding the attention-based MIL pooling (Bag-level MINN+attention"), the GCNs (Bag-level MINN+GNN+attention), and the instance-level supervision (Bag-level MINN+GNN+ attention+all instance supervised). In the implementation of Bag-level MINN+GNN+ attention+all instance supervised, all instances of the positive bags were labelled as positive.

In the ablation studies, we randomly selected 79 MH and 99 CAKUT patients as a training data set, random 45 subjects from the remaining dataset were used as a validation data set. This procedure was repeated twice to estimate the classification performance of different versions of the proposed method. Their classification results are summarized in Table 1, demonstrating that GCNs, the attention-based MIL pooling, and the instance-level supervision based on instances with reliable labels could improve the MIL classification performance. Particularly, these results also indicated that the instance-level supervision based on all instance might be affected by the instance label instability problem [12].

We further evaluated our method and compared it with state-of-the-art MIL methods, including CNN based instance level classification with max MIL pooling (minet) [9], embedded-space based deep MIL method with mean (Minet+mean) MIL pooling [10], as well as embedded-space based deep MIL with an attention-based MIL pooling (Gated-Attention) [11]. All the deep MIL methods under comparison had the same CNNs with the same numbers of parameters. In the minet, we labelled all instances of the positive bags as positive instances. The classification performance of these methods were estimated using 5-fold cross-validation. All the classification results are summarized in Table 2. These results further demonstrated that our method could improve the classification performance of the state-of-the-art MIL methods.

Table 2. Comparison results of different MIL methods (mean±std)

Method	Accuracy	Sensitivity	Specificity
Minet	0.6488 ± 0.0852	0.5917 ± 0.1037	0.7143 ± 0.1683
Minet	0.8044 ± 0.0656	0.8250 ± 0.1229	0.7809 ± 0.1372
Gated-Attention	0.8222 ± 0.0471	0.8083 ± 0.0228	0.8381 ± 0.0865
Proposed	0.8489 ± 0.0365	0.8582 ± 0.0697	0.8381 ± 0.0865

Finally, we adopted Grad-CAM to identify informative image regions for the classification [15]. Figure 3 shows Grad-CAM maps of two randomly selected testing subjects with CAKUT. Particularly, instances with relatively larger weights learned by the attention-based MIL pooling are shown from left to right, indicating that our method could capture clinically meaningful image features.

Example Subject 1

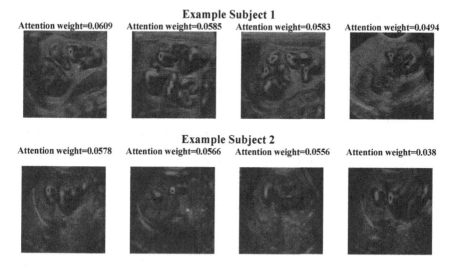

Example Subject 2

Fig. 3. Two examples of the multi-instance Grad-CAM maps of abnormal subjects with relatively lager attention weights. The largest weight across all test subjects was about 0.06.

4   Conclusions

In this study, we develop a novel multi-instance deep learning method to build a robust classifier to aid kidney disease diagnosis using ultrasound imaging. Our method is built upon recent advance in deep MIL on the embedded-space [10, 11] with novel components, including the GCNs to optimize the instance-level features learned by CNNs and the integrated instance-level and bag-level supervision to improve the classification. Extensive ablation studies and comparison experiments have demonstrated that our method could improve state-of-the-art deep MIL methods for the kidney disease diagnosis. Our future work will be devoted to automatic network architecture optimization and extensive validation of the proposed method based on different data sets.

Acknowledgements. This work was supported in part by the National Institutes of Health (DK117297 and DK114786); the National Center for Advancing Translational Sciences of the National Institutes of Health (UL1TR001878); the National Natural Science Foundation of China (61772220 and 61473296); the Key Program for International S&T Cooperation Projects of China (2016YFE0121200); the Hubei Province Technological Innovation Major Project (2017AAA017 and 2018ACA135); the Institute for Translational Medicine and Therapeutics' (ITMAT) Transdisciplinary Program in Translational Medicine and Therapeutics, and the China Scholarship Council.

References

1. Cost, G.A., Merguerian, P.A., Cheerasarn, S.P., Shortliffe, L.M.D.: Sonographic renal parenchymal and pelvicaliceal areas: new quantitative parameters for renal sonographic followup. J. Urol. **156**, 725–729 (1996)
2. Sharma, K., Virmani, J.: A decision support system for classification of normal and medical renal disease using ultrasound images: a decision support system for medical renal diseases. Int. J. Ambient Comput. Intell. **8**, 52–69 (2017)
3. Subramanya, M.B., Kumar, V., Mukherjee, S., Saini, M.: SVM-based CAC system for B-mode kidney ultrasound images. J. Digit. Imaging **28**, 448–458 (2015)
4. Liu, S., et al.: Deep learning in medical ultrasound analysis: a review. Engineering **5**, 261–275 (2019)
5. Yin, S., et al.: Subsequent boundary distance regression and pixelwise classification networks for automatic kidney segmentation in ultrasound images. arXiv preprint arXiv: 1811.04815 (2018)
6. Yin, S., et al.: Fully-automatic segmentation of kidneys in clinical ultrasound images using a boundary distance regression network. In: 2019 IEEE 16th International Symposium on Biomedical Imaging (ISBI 2019), pp. 1741–1744 (2019)
7. Amores, J.: Multiple instance classification: review, taxonomy and comparative study. Artif. Intell. **201**, 81–105 (2013)
8. Ramon, J., De Raedt, L.: Multi instance neural networks (2000)
9. Zhou, Z.-H., Zhang, M.-L.: Neural networks for multi-instance learning. In: Proceedings of the International Conference on Intelligent Information Technology, Beijing, China, pp. 455–459 (2002)
10. Wang, X., Yan, Y., Tang, P., Bai, X., Liu, W.: Revisiting multiple instance neural networks. Pattern Recogn. **74**, 15–24 (2018)
11. Ilse, M., Tomczak, J., Welling, M.: Attention-based deep multiple instance learning. In: Jennifer, D., Andreas, K. (eds.) Proceedings of the 35th International Conference on Machine Learning, PMLR, Proceedings of Machine Learning Research, vol. 80, pp. 2127–2136 (2018)
12. Cheplygina, V., Sørensen, L., Tax, D.M.J., de Bruijne, M., Loog, M.: Label stability in multiple instance learning. In: Navab, N., Hornegger, J., Wells, W.M., Frangi, A.F. (eds.) MICCAI 2015. LNCS, vol. 9349, pp. 539–546. Springer, Cham (2015). https://doi.org/10.1007/978-3-319-24553-9_66
13. Goodfellow, I., Bengio, Y., Courville, A.: Deep Learning. MIT Press, Cambridge (2016)
14. Kipf, T.N., Welling, M.: Semi-supervised classification with graph convolutional networks. arXiv preprint arXiv:1609.02907 (2016)
15. Selvaraju, R.R., Cogswell, M., Das, A., Vedantam, R., Parikh, D., Batra, D.: Grad-CAM: visual explanations from deep networks via gradient-based localization. arXiv:1610.02391 (2016)

Data Augmentation from Sketch

Debora Gil[1], Antonio Esteban-Lansaque[1], Sebastian Stefaniga[2],
Mihail Gaianu[2], and Carles Sanchez[1(✉)]

[1] Computer Vision Center, Computer Science Deptartment, UAB, Barcelona, Spain
{debora,csanchez}@cvc.uab.es
[2] Computer Science Deptartment, West University of Timisoara, Timişoara, Romania

Abstract. State of the art machine learning methods need huge amounts of data with unambiguous annotations for their training. In the context of medical imaging this is, in general, a very difficult task due to limited access to clinical data, the time required for manual annotations and variability across experts. Simulated data could serve for data augmentation provided that its appearance was comparable to the actual appearance of intra-operative acquisitions. Generative Adversarial Networks (GANs) are a powerful tool for artistic style transfer, but lack a criteria for selecting epochs ensuring also preservation of intra-operative content.

We propose a multi-objective optimization strategy for a selection of cycleGAN epochs ensuring a mapping between virtual images and the intra-operative domain preserving anatomical content. Our approach has been applied to simulate intra-operative bronchoscopic videos and chest CT scans from virtual sketches generated using simple graphical primitives.

Keywords: Data augmentation · cycleGANs · Multi-objective optimization

1 Introduction

Medical imaging applications are challenging for machine learning methods due to the difficulty to generate reliable ground truth and the limited size of annotated databases. Data augmentation [1] has become a standard procedure to improve the training process. Data augmentation schemes increase the number of training samples by simple transformations (like translation, rotation, flip and scale) of the original dataset images. However, the diversity that can be gained from such modifications of the images is relatively small and introduces correlations in training data.

Virtual images obtained from computer simulations could be used to train classifiers and validate image processing methods if their appearance was comparable (in texture and color) to the actual appearance of intra-operative data. We consider that style transfer could be used to endow virtual simulated data with the content and texture of intra-operative scans using modern techniques for artistic style transfer.

© Springer Nature Switzerland AG 2019
H. Greenspan et al. (Eds.): CLIP 2019/UNSURE 2019, LNCS 11840, pp. 155–162, 2019.
https://doi.org/10.1007/978-3-030-32689-0_16

Recent works [2,3] have shown the power of Generative Adversarial Networks (GANs) for artistic style transfer. These methods generate stylized images comparing image feature representations extracted from pre-computed convolutional neural networks. A main challenge is the generation of pairs with similar content ensuring preservation of anatomical features. To avoid pairings, new approaches like [3] use GANs to transform images from one domain A (like virtual simulations) into a domain B (like interventional videos). The novelty of [3] is that a cyclic term is added in order to make the domain transfer bijective ($A \to B \to A$ and $B \to A \to B$). Although this endows maps with some content preservation, a main challenge [4] is the selection of the epochs most suitable for a given problem. Due to the oscillating behavior of adversarial training, most of the cases this is done manually.

Recently, several works using GANs for medical data augmentation have been proposed [5–8]. These works lack for a criteria to chose the best trained epoch depending on the target task. As it is stated in [8], rigorous performance evaluation of GANs is an important research area, since is not clear how to quantitatively evaluate generative models [9]. In particular, when using statistical methods, like [3], aside probability distributions among pixels, their geometric relations related to anatomical content should also be taken into account. Such geometrical content should be considered in the definition of virtual data and it might not be easy to model in case of complex multi-organ scans. The most usual approach is to use anatomies already segmented, which might imply access to large amount of annotated data for generating new cases.

In this work, we propose a multi-objective optimization approach based on the Pareto front [10] to select the cycleGAN epoch achieving the best compromise between content preservation and style transfer. As a proof-of-concept, our multi-objective cycleGAN has been applied to simulate bronchoscopic videos and chest CT scans from synthetic models of the anatomy sketched using graphical primitives. As far as we know this is the first work generating several anatomies from simple geometrical models.

2   Multi-objective cycleGAN

Given two domains $Virtual$, V, and $Real$, R, style transfer learns two (bijective) maps (G_r, G_v) from one domain onto the other one:

$$G_r : Virtual \to Real \quad G_v : Real \to Virtual \tag{1}$$

with the map composition $G_r(G_v)$ and $G_v(G_r)$ being the identity on each domain. Following [3], maps are given by auto-encoders trained to optimize:

$$\ell(G_r, G_v, D_r, D_v) = \ell_{\mathbf{GAN}}(G_v, G_r, D_r, D_v, V, R) + \lambda \ell_{\mathbf{cyc}}(G_v, G_r) \tag{2}$$

The term $\ell_{\mathbf{GAN}}$ measures how good are G_v, G_r transferring images from one domain to the other one, while $\ell_{\mathbf{cyc}}$ is a "cycle consistency loss" introduced to force bijective mappings.

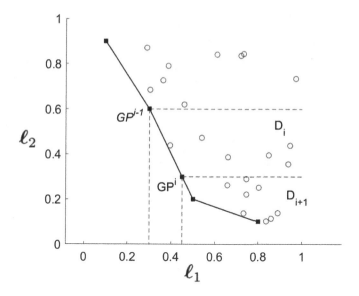

Fig. 1. Pareto front of cycle-GAN 2-objective optimization.

The minimization problem is solved by adversarial training as:

$$G_r^*, G_v^* = \min_{G_r, G_v} \left(\max_{D_r, D_v} \ell(G_r, G_v, D_r, D_v) \right) \tag{3}$$

In this manner, G_r^* and G_v^* are optimized so that G_r, G_v minimize (2) while the adversarial D_r, D_v maximize it. These conditions (minimize while maximizing at the same time) might be in conflict considered into a single optimization process and might hinder the convergence of the training back-propagation.

We propose to consider separately the optimization of each of the terms in ℓ and pose adversarial training as a multi-objective optimization [10] problem:

$$\begin{aligned} G_r^*, G_v^* &= \min_{G_r, G_v} (\ell_1, \ell_2) = \min_{G_r, G_v} (\ell_{\mathbf{cyc}}, \ell_{\mathbf{GAN}}) \\ &= \min_{G_r, G_v} (\ell_{\mathbf{cyc}}(G_r, G_v), \max_{D_r, D_v} \ell_{\mathbf{GAN}}(G_v, G_r, D_r, D_v)) \end{aligned} \tag{4}$$

The solution to (4) is computed from the Pareto front [10] consisting in the set of dominating configurations that outperform in any of the objectives without degrading at least one of the other ones. For this two-objective problem we compute an approximation to the Pareto front from back-propagation epochs as follows.

Let $\boldsymbol{G}^k := (G_r^k, G_v^k)$ be the transformation maps at the k-th epoch and $\boldsymbol{GP} = (\boldsymbol{GP}^i)_{i=1}^{NP}$ be the set of epochs belonging to the Pareto front. Such Pareto maps can be iteratively computed from the values of the objective functions as:

$$\boldsymbol{GP}^i := \min_{\boldsymbol{G}^i \in \boldsymbol{D}_i} (\ell_{\mathbf{cyc}}(\boldsymbol{G}^i)) \tag{5}$$

for D_1 the set of maps for all epochs and D_i, $i > 2$, the set of maps dominating GP^{i-1}. In our case, $G^i \in D_i$ if it satisfies the following conditions:

$$1.\ \ell_{\mathrm{cyc}}(G^i) > \ell_{\mathrm{cyc}}(GP^{i-1}) \quad 2.\ \ell_{\mathrm{GAN}}(G^i) < \ell_{\mathrm{GAN}}(GP^{i-1})$$

Figure 1 shows the Pareto front associated to the two-objective problem given by (4) with the dashed lines enclosing the region that includes the set of epochs that dominate a given GP^{i-1}. The pairs of function values $(\ell_{\mathrm{cyc}}(GP^i), \ell_{\mathrm{GAN}}(GP^i))$, $GP^i \in GP$, given by the two objectives evaluated at the Pareto front are shown in solid squares joined with a solid line.

We note that, by construction, our approximation to the Pareto front contains the epoch achieving the minimum of (2). Due to adversarial training, this epoch might be an early one prone to have high ℓ_{GAN}. In order to select Pareto epochs producing style images with higher real appearance, a clustering or threshold on Pareto epochs ℓ_{GAN} values could be considered as filtering post-processing.

3   Experiments

The proposed multi-objective cycleGAN has been applied to simulate intra-operative virtual bronchoscopies and chest CT scans. For each modality, a different cycleGAN was trained using intra-operative data and tested in virtual sketches of the anatomy observed in each modality. Each CycleGAN was trained for 200 epochs.

3.1   Intra-operative Virtual Bronchoscopies

For this experiment we trained a cycleGAN on a set of 5 ultrathin intra-operative recordings (defining the set of images of the *Real* domain, R) and 5 virtual bronchoscopies (defining the set of images of the *Virtual* domain, V). Intra-operative videos were acquired during biopsy interventions at Hospital Bellvitge (Barcelona, Spain) using an Olympus Exera III HD Ultrathin videobroncho-scope. Virtual bronchoscopies were generated using an own developed software from CT scans acquired for different patients with an Aquilion^{TM} ONE (Toshiba Medical Systems, Otawara, Japan) using slice thickness and interval of 0.5 and 0.4 mm respectively. For each intra-operative video or virtual simulation, we randomly selected 500 images for training cycleGAN from scratch.

In order to validate our proposal, we generated 10 sequences using sketches of airways in bronchoscopic frames. Sketches of airways were produced using elliptical shapes of different sizes and eccentricity and considering several con-figurations in number and disposition in the image. For each configuration, a sequence of affine transformations was applied to simulate bronchoscopic navi-gation.

Figure 2 plots the two cost functions for all epochs with the 35 Pareto epochs in black crosses. The epochs selected for these experiment are shown in squares, green ones for epochs on the Pareto front, red ones, otherwise. We have selected 2 epochs not belonging to the Pareto front, one (epoch 80) far from it, another one (epoch 70) close to it. The epochs selected on the Pareto front are the boundary ones (199, 21, which is the one achieving the minimum value of (2)) and the epoch (122) closest to epoch 70.

Figure 3 shows a mosaic of representative sketches and their augmentation using the 5 epochs. For each sketch, we show consecutive frames to check the stability of the augmented images. Images obtained from Pareto epochs have a green frame, red otherwise. As it can be seen, the appearance of images generated with Pareto front epochs are more stable and keep better texture. Also brightness, color and the shape of holes are more realistic. Epoch 21 artifacts on image boundary and lack of texture can be attributed to an early stage of cycleGAN training. It is worth noticing that images generated with epochs not belonging to the Pareto front (like epoch 80) present an unstable anatomy with new holes that were not in the sketches.

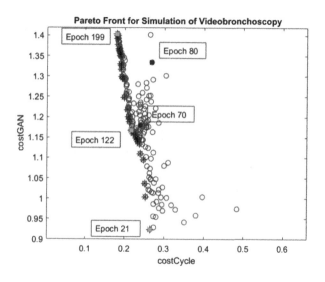

Fig. 2. Pareto front for Intra-operative virtual bronchoscopies. (Color figure online)

3.2   Chest CT Scans

For this experiment we trained a cycleGAN on a set of 11 chest CT volumes (defining the *Real* domain) and their segmentation (defining the *Virtual* domain) of the main lung structures. CT scans were acquired in inspiration with an Aquilion^{TM} ONE (Toshiba Medical Systems, Otawara, Japan) using slice thickness and interval of 0.5 and 0.4 mm respectively. Segmentations included the body, lungs, pulmonary vessels and airways and were computed using an own-designed software. Each volume (original CT scan and its segmentation)

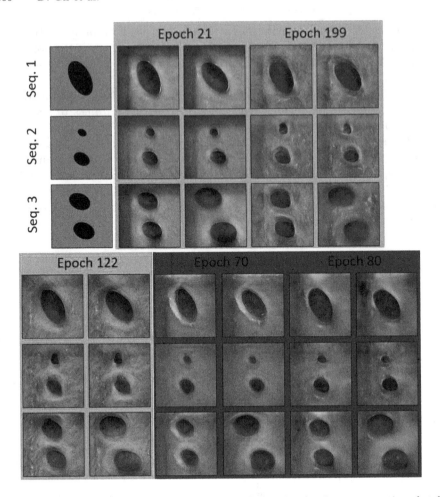

Fig. 3. Generated intra-operative virtual bronchoscopies for 3 representative sketch sequences: images from Pareto front epochs in green frame and images from non-Pareto epochs in red one. (Color figure online)

was uniformly sampled in 250 short axis planes covering the whole volume of lungs for training cycleGAN from scratch.

A total number of 10 anatomical sketches were generated using 3D graphical primitives for each lung structure. Body was modelled with a cylinder, lungs with ellipsoids and, both, vessels and airways were modelled as tubular structures with several branching levels. The thickness of the tubes was set depending on the level to account for different lumen sizes. To endow sketches with more realistic geometry, the cardiac and abdominal cavities were also modelled using ellipsoids. The ranges for primitives sizes were statistically learned from segmented CTs. For each sketched anatomy 250 short axis planes were sampled for testing.

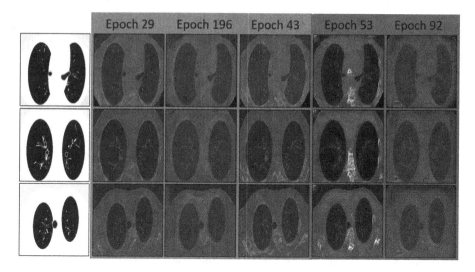

Fig. 4. Generated CT virtual scans for 3 representative (distal, mid, basal) sketches: images from Pareto front epochs in green frame and images from non-Pareto epochs in red one. (Color figure online)

In this case, the Pareto front had 7 epochs. As in the previous experiment, we selected the Pareto boundary epochs (196 and the least cost 29), two epochs not belonging to the Pareto front (epoch 92 far from it and epoch 53 close to it) and the Pareto epoch (43) closest to epoch 53. Figure 4 shows a mosaic of representative sketches and their augmentation using these 5 epochs. Image frame colors are like in Fig. 3. As before, images generated with epochs not belonging to the Pareto front present different artifacts, like a stripe pattern (epoch 92), lack of texture in lungs (epoch 53) and bright structures in the body (epoch 53). Meanwhile, images generated with Pareto epochs keep a stable appearance similar to the one of a chest CT scan.

4   Conclusions

In this paper, we propose a generative algorithm based on cycleGANs to produce synthetic medical data from simple graphical primitives roughly approximating the anatomical structure of organs. In particular, we present a novel multi-objective analysis of cycleGAN training epochs for the selection of epochs achieving the best compromise between generation and discrimination.

Models have been tested in synthetic videobronchoscopy sequences and chest CT scans computed using simple graphical primitives. Visual inspection of this proof-of-concept indicates that networks might admit a training on limited amount of data thanks to a numerical analysis of the back-propagation scheme. Results also indicate that the epochs selected by our multi-objective approach have a good generalization power in testing on data with geometrical structure different from the one of training data.

These results encourage further investigation of the performance of using sketches (easy to generate without large gathering of medical data) for training networks and augment sets using more realistic anatomies computed from few medical scans.

Acknowledgments. The research leading to these results has received funding from the European Union's Horizon 2020 research and innovation programme under the Marie Sklodowska-Curie grant agreement No 712949 (TECNIOspring PLUS) and from the Agency for Business Competitiveness of the Government of Catalonia. Work supported by Spanish Projects FIS-G64384969, Generalitat de Catalunya, 2017-SGR-1624 and CERCA-Programme. D. Gil is a Serra Hunter fellow. The Titan X Pascal used for this research was donated by the NVIDIA Corporation.

References

1. Krizhevsky, A., Sutskever, I., Hinton, G.E.: Imagenet classification with deep convolutional neural networks. In: Advances in Neural Information Processing Systems, pp. 1097–1105 (2012)
2. Johnson, J., Alahi, A., Fei-Fei, L.: Perceptual losses for real-time style transfer and super-resolution. In: Leibe, B., Matas, J., Sebe, N., Welling, M. (eds.) ECCV 2016. LNCS, vol. 9906, pp. 694–711. Springer, Cham (2016). https://doi.org/10.1007/978-3-319-46475-6_43
3. Zhu, J.-Y., Park, T., Isola, P., Efros, A.A.: Unpaired image-to-image translation using cycle-consistent adversarial networks. arXiv preprint arXiv:1703.10593 (2017)
4. Radford, A., Metz, L., Chintala, S.: Unsupervised representation learning with deep convolutional generative adversarial networks. arXiv preprint arXiv:1511.06434 (2015)
5. Frid-Adar, M., Klang, E., Amitai, M., Goldberger, J., Greenspan, H.: Synthetic data augmentation using GAN for improved liver lesion classification. In: 2018 IEEE 15th International Symposium on Biomedical Imaging (ISBI 2018), pp. 289–293. IEEE (2018)
6. Shin, H.-C., et al.: Medical image synthesis for data augmentation and anonymization using generative adversarial networks. In: Gooya, A., Goksel, O., Oguz, I., Burgos, N. (eds.) SASHIMI 2018. LNCS, vol. 11037, pp. 1–11. Springer, Cham (2018). https://doi.org/10.1007/978-3-030-00536-8_1
7. Frid-Adar, M., Diamant, I., Klang, E., Amitai, M., Goldberger, J., Greenspan, H.: Gan-based synthetic medical image augmentation for increased CNN performance in liver lesion classification. Neurocomputing **321**, 321–331 (2018)
8. Calimeri, F., Marzullo, A., Stamile, C., Terracina, G.: Biomedical data augmentation using generative adversarial neural networks. In: Lintas, A., Rovetta, S., Verschure, P.F.M.J., Villa, A.E.P. (eds.) ICANN 2017. LNCS, vol. 10614, pp. 626–634. Springer, Cham (2017). https://doi.org/10.1007/978-3-319-68612-7_71
9. Goodfellow, I., Bengio, Y., Courville, A.: Deep Learning. MIT Press, Cambridge (2016)
10. Miettinen, K.: Nonlinear Multiobjective Optimization, vol. 12. Springer, New York (2012). https://doi.org/10.1007/978-1-4615-5563-6

An Automated CNN-based 3D Anatomical Landmark Detection Method to Facilitate Surface-Based 3D Facial Shape Analysis

Ruobing Huang[1(✉)], Michael Suttie[2], and J. Alison Noble[1]

[1] Institute of Biomedical Engineering, University of Oxford, Oxford, UK
ruobing.huang@eng.ox.ac.uk
[2] Nuffield Department of Women's and Reproductive Health,
University of Oxford, Oxford, UK

Abstract. Maternal alcohol consumption during pregnancy can lead to a wide range of physical and neurodevelopmental problems, collectively known as fetal alcohol spectrum disorders (FASD). In many cases, diagnosis is heavily reliant on the recognition of a set of characteristic facial features, which can be subtle and difficult to objectively identify. To provide an automated and objective way to quantify these features, this paper proposes to take advantage of high-resolution 3D facial scans collected from a high-risk population. We present a method to automatically localize anatomical landmarks on each face, and align them to a standard space. Subsequent surface-based morphology analysis or anatomical measurements demands that such a method is both accurate and robust.

The CNN-based model uses a novel differentiable spatial to numerical transform (DSNT) layer that could transform spatial activation to numerical values directly, which enables end-to-end training. Experiments reveal that the inserted layer helps to boost the performance and achieves sub-pixel level accuracy.

Keywords: FASD · Landmark detection · 3D facial analysis

1 Introduction

Maternal drinking in pregnancy can result in fetal central nervous system damage, and fetal and young child growth deficiency, cranio-facial abnormalities, learning disabilities and functional impairments [1]. The range of phenotypes varies greatly in severity and presentation, largely dependent on the level, pattern, and timing of maternal alcohol consumption therefore termed as: fetal alcohol spectrum disorder (FASD). The prevalence of FASD has been documented as high as 13.5%–20.8% in some regions, and produces an immense burden to families and society [1].

© Springer Nature Switzerland AG 2019
H. Greenspan et al. (Eds.): CLIP 2019/UNSURE 2019, LNCS 11840, pp. 163–171, 2019.
https://doi.org/10.1007/978-3-030-32689-0_17

Formal diagnosis at the earliest possible stage is paramount, as it allows early intervention and reduces the risk of secondary disabilities [1]. However, the diagnosis of FASD is particularly challenging due to the inconspicuous brain malformations in young children, unreliable reports of maternal alcohol usage, and misdiagnosis of syndromes with similar characteristics. Recognition of the most severe form, fetal alcohol syndrome (FAS), is reliant on the identification of 3 cardinal facial features: short palpebral fissure length (PFL), a smooth philtrum and a thin upper lip. Current methods for facial assessment are necessarily subjective and vary between clinicians. For example, clinicians score the lip and the philtrum using a 5-point Likert scale for visual comparison (Fig. 1) [1]. To measure PFL, some clinicians place a ruler on the subjects' face, whereas others use a semi-automated 2D software. Both methods for facial evaluation involve subjectivity, and accuracy can be influenced by the skill and experience of the clinician. Some prior studies have pointed out that PFL obtained in 3D can be more stable while they relied on manually annotated 3D landmarks [2].

To overcome these difficulties, we propose an automated method to detect 3D anatomical landmarks to calculate anthropometric measurements and facilitate surface-based 3D shape analysis. Using a differential spatial-to-numerical layer, the trained model is compact and predicts the target coordinates directly without the need for post-processing or fully-connected layers. To the best of our knowledge, this is the first time that a fully automatic method has been proposed to assist FASD diagnosis using 3D facial form.

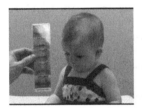 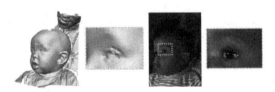

Fig. 1. FAS diagnosis. (Image credit:https://www.youtube. com/watch?v=044Zxy3_0u8.)

Fig. 2. 3D mesh and the corresponding texture map (zoomed in the eye region). Key part of face is masked to protect privacy.

2   Related Works

Before discussing the related literature and the proposed method, we first introduce our dataset as it is different from commonly used medical imaging data. The dataset was collected using a static stereo-photogrammetric camera system produced by 3DMD. By simultaneously taking photos using two cameras with fixed positions, the system is able to reconstruct a dense 3D surface. Each facial scan consists of a 3D mesh (Fig. 2) and two 2D photographs (also referred to as texture maps). The 3D mesh is defined by an OBJ file where the link between each polygon face and the corresponding texture map regions is also included for color rendering. Each 3D mesh consists of more than 30,000 vertices representing surface geometry, and all texture maps are resized to 256 × 256 pixels. For this study, 3D images of an ethnically admixed population of unexposed and prenatal alcohol-exposed infants at 1–12 months were used from the Prenatal Alcohol and SIDS and Stillbirth (PASS) Network in Stellenbosch, South Africa (n = 777, Fig. 3). Among them, 305 are alcohol-exposed cases. The dataset was randomly separated into training (n = 622) and test (n = 155) sets. 20 reliable landmarks were manually annotated in 3D on each face by an expert, and were projected to each corresponding 2D texture map as training labels for the CNN models.

Manual 3D landmark placement is a tedious and potentially error-prone task, but is often a necessity for 3D shape analysis. Literature is abundant in detecting landmarks in 2D images and relatively new in 3D. We refer the interested reader to [3] for a recent review. Detecting 3D landmarks automatically is difficult as processing a high-resolution 3D mesh is non-trivial. There are also some successful works in computer vision that process 3D points cloud or meshes directly [4–6]. However, these approaches mainly addressed classification or segmentation. More importantly, they usually require a large dataset to train those complicate models which is not available in our case. Another key observation is that the surface of the mesh is less well-defined than the corresponding texture map in regions of complex geometry such as the eye corners and eyebrows (Fig. 2). Therefore, we approach the problem by detecting landmarks on the 2D texture map and propagate the results back to 3D for further analysis.

Besides the common challenges faced in detecting 2D landmarks, e.g. large appearance variations, environmental conditions changes, and occlusions caused by extreme head poses, our task has additional challenges. The age group and ethnic background of the subjects is substantially different from the web-collected datasets (e.g. CelebA) widely used in computer vision. Our preliminary experiments showed that models trained on these datasets failed to detect the face in our dataset constantly (up to 24%)[1]. Further, the annotation of the landmarks is performed in 3D, thus the training labels of our 2D detection model are obtained by projecting these 3D points on the 2D texture map using UV unwrapping. As a result, the location of the same landmark (e.g. the outer corner of the left eye) could appear at very different locations on the texture map and the

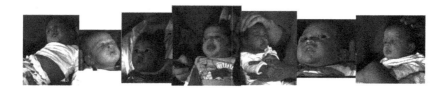

Fig. 3. Examples of subjects' texture maps contained in this challenging dataset.

---

[1] This is echoed by an extensive study in face recognition [7], which showed CV models could fail on nearly 35% on darker skinned females.

number of annotated landmarks on each photo is uncertain. The addressed task requires quantitative accuracy, and therefore needs specialized design.

Among existing landmark detection methods [8,9], some of the most successful ones leveraged the power of convolution neural networks (CNNs), and could be mainly divided into two groups: (1) coordinate regression by attaching a fully connected layers at the end; and (2) matching synthetic heatmaps that are generated by placing a 2D Gaussian at the target location. The first approach can be trained using the raw labels while some valuable spatial information is lost during flattening. The heatmap matching approach takes advantage of the translation invariant characteristics of CNNs as neurons can be activated anywhere in the visual field and scored the highest accuracy in many benchmarks. However, during inference, the coordinates are derived by extracting the brightest pixel in the output, which typically involves a non-differential argmax operation. As a result, there is a disconnect between the training loss function and the evaluation metrics that might lead to convergence at a sub-optimal minimum.

3   Method

Figure 4 shows a schematic of the analysis pipeline. During test time, two unseen texture maps are individually passed into a CNN model for landmark detection. The results are then combined and projected back to automatically label the corresponding 3D mesh. Using the detected set of landmarks we can calculate relevant anatomical measurements, and utilize tools for surface-based shape analysis. By doing so, individual and group dysmorphism can be quantified by calculating the normalized surface-based differences against controls [10].

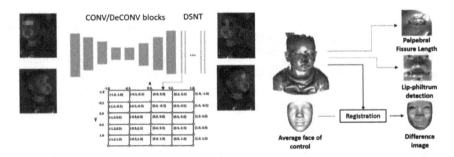

Fig. 4. Schematic of the proposed pipeline. The texture maps are passed into the CNN model which consists of several convolutional (CONV) and deCONV blocks (blue) and DNST layers (grey) that yield landmark locations (red dots) directly. The results are propagated to 3D to produce clinical measurements and morphological analysis. (Color figure online)

DSNT Layer. The key idea of the proposed CNN model is the incorporation of a novel layer. As discussed before, the heatmap matching method has one disadvantage that could hamper performance: a gap between the target metric and the optimized loss function. The solution for this boils down to find a differentiable way to extract coordinates from heatmap-like activations.

Following [11], we insert a DSNT layer at the end of our CNN model. The key insight here is that the value of each pixel $p_{i,j} \in \mathcal{P}$ in the predicted heatmap $\mathcal{P}$ essentially indicates the likelihood of that pixel being the target landmark $C = \{x, y\}$. In other words, if we first normalize $\mathcal{P}$ to $\hat{\mathcal{P}} = \frac{\mathcal{P}}{\sum \mathcal{P}}$ such that for $\hat{p}_{i,j} \in \hat{\mathcal{P}}$ it satisfies that $\sum_{i,j} \hat{p}_{i,j} = 1$, $\hat{\mathcal{P}}$ could be interpreted as the probability distribution of the location of the target landmark. The expected value of the target coordinate distribution can then be calculated as the inner product of the normalized heatmap $\hat{\mathcal{P}}$ and the same size coordinate mesh-grid. More formally, given the size of final activation map $\hat{\mathcal{P}}$ is $H \times W$, we construct a 2D mesh-grid that satisfy: $X_{i,j} = \frac{2i-1-H}{H}, Y_{i,j} = \frac{2j-1-W}{W}$. The value of each pixel is proportional to its distance from the origin in a specific direction and ranges from $[-1, 1]$ (Fig. 4). The expectation of the target coordinates $C = \{x, y\}$, could be derived as:

$$E(C(x,y)) = \{< \hat{P}, X >, < \hat{P}, Y >\}, \tag{1}$$

where $< \cdot >$ denotes the Frobenius inner product operation. As this operation is differentiable and fast to compute, it enables the model to learn from the ground truth (GT) coordinates directly. This meshgrid can be easily constructed and hard-coded into the layer before training, introducing no additional parameters.

Inserting the DSNT layer naively, however, does not guarantee good results. Two main issues are: (1) there is no constraint to penalize the presence of false-positive clutters - the appearance of normalized heatmaps could vary dramatically yet produce the same prediction; (2) limited supervision is provided to update the parameters of the whole network. To address both issues, a regularization term is appended to the loss function to penalize the spread of activations. This is achieved by controlling the variance of the modeled coordinate distribution $Var(C(x,y))$, computed as:

$$Var(C_v) = E(C_v)^2 - [E(C_v)]^2 = < \hat{P}, C_v^2 > - [< \hat{P}, C_v >]^2,$$

for each component $C_v \in x, y$. Given a variance controlling threshold φ, the overall variance could be computed as:

$$\mathcal{L}_{var} = \sum_{C_v \in x,y} (Var(C_v) - \varphi)^2 \tag{2}$$

The overall loss function is:

$$\mathcal{L}_{var} = \mathcal{L}_{coor} + \beta \mathcal{L}_{var}, \tag{3}$$

where β is a hyper-parameter to control the weight of the regularizer and $\mathcal{L}_{coor}$ is the Euclidean distance between the ground truth and the prediction.

Backward Projection. Detecting facial landmarks from 2D images is an ill-posed problem. However, we can use the 2D results to infer the landmark locations in 3D utilizing the connection between the texture map and the polygon surface. Specifically, we unwrap the 3D mesh on the whole texture map, then find the 3D polygon face that is the closet to the detected landmarks. As each face mesh consists of thousands of small surfaces, the area of each polygon surface is very small and could be regarded as a point. Therefore, the geometric center of this polygon is a good approximation of the target landmark location in 3D (Fig. 5).

The derived 3D landmarks are then used to calculate PFL and utilized for subsequent surface-based analysis using dense surface modelling (DSM). The derived DSM, in turn, enables atypical facial morphology detection (e.g. lower-right in Fig. 4) and helps FAS-control discrimination.

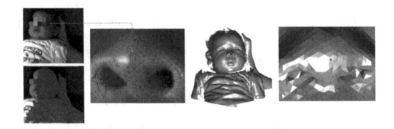

Fig. 5. Example of the 2D to 3D projection process. The nose tip is detected (red) on the 2D images. The 3D mesh is unwrap on the texture map (plotted as grey line). The closet 3D polygon surface to the landmark is found and its center is used to approximate the 3D position of the nose tip (plotted on the white 3D mesh). (Color figure online)

4   Experiments

To demonstrate the effectiveness of the DSNT layer, we tested two comparative models. (1) Regression-based model ($\mathcal{RB}$). It uses a classical CNN model that consists of interlaced convolution (CONV) and down-sampling layers, followed by a fully-connected layer that predicts the target coordinates directly. (2) Synthetic heatmap matching. This method is tested with two different CNN models. The vanilla model (denoted as $\mathcal{HM_V}$) contains a down-sampling and up-sampling stream, the model branched out in the end into 20 prediction layers to predict the location heatmap of each landmark respectively. The second model follows the well-known work of [9], two vanilla CNNs are concatenated together into a hourglass-like model. This model (denoted as $\mathcal{HM_H}$) can capture information from different scales more freely which has proved to be helpful in landmark localization.

Implementation Details. The backbone of the tested CNN models contained four CONV block and down-sampling layers, while $\mathcal{HM_V}, \mathcal{HM_H}$ also have symmetrical up-sampling layers. A kernel of size 3×3 was used across the whole model. The numbers of feature channels for CONV layers are 8, 16, 32, and 64 for all remaining layers. Model training was done end-to-end via the Adam optimizer.

5   Results and Conclusion

Qualitative results of our model are shown in Fig. 6. The upper-right example in Fig. 6 is a particularly interesting case, as the subject is difficult to differentiate from the background due to the lighting conditions. However, the model was able to locate facial key-points accurately. Overall, the figure shows that our model is robust to appearance variations caused by extreme head pose (upper-left) facial expression (e.g. closed eyes in the upper middle and upper-right) and different ethnic background (lower-right and lower-middle).

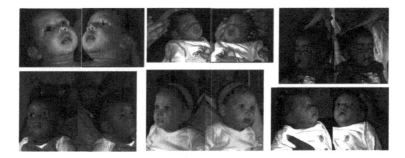

Fig. 6. Predicted landmarks (red) on the test set. The images are resized to fit the page while the aspect ratio is kept to avoid distortion during visualization. (Color figure online)

The localization accuracy was evaluated by calculating the Euclidean distance between the ground truth (GT) and the predictions in 2D (Table. 1). It can be seen that our model has the best accuracy despite its smaller size. $\mathcal{RB}$ has a large error, which may result from the fact that the GT landmark have large location variations therefore the model is confused in training. It is also interesting to see that $\mathcal{HM_V}$ outperformed $\mathcal{HM_S}$ in landmark detection by a small margin. This might be caused by overfitting as the $\mathcal{HM_S}$ has a more complex network structure that requires more training data. A light-weight model is therefore memory-efficient and well-suited for our task.

The 2D detection results are propagated to the corresponding 3D meshes to obtain the 3D coordinates of each landmark. As children have fast growing trajectories, their faces can have very different sizes. To better evaluate the results, we adopt the popular normalized error metric:

$$norm\_err = \frac{1}{N} \sum_{i}^{N} \frac{|d_i - g_i|_2}{|g_{re} - g_{le}|_2}, \tag{4}$$

while N is the number of evaluated landmarks, $|\cdot|_2$ is the Euclidean distance between two points[2], d_i and g_i are the predicted coordinates and the GT for the i_{th} landmark. $|g_{re} - g_{le}|_2$ is the inter-ocular distance: the Euclidean distance between the center of the two eyes. Note that we only use this metric in 3D as the annotations for both of the eyes do not co-exist in a single 2D image (see how the eyes are annotated in Fig. 4). The accuracy results of our model is comparable to those reported on computer vision datasets [3], further proving the effectiveness of our model (Table 1). Table 1 also reports the reliability of the automated generated PFL measurements. Our model has the smallest deviation from the GT (calculated based on manual annotations) while the $\mathcal{RB}$ performed the worst. It should be pointed out the PFL derived from 3D meshes could be more reliable than from the current clinical method (placing a ruler against the subject face). The promotion of such a model might help automate and standardize this process.

Furthermore, the method allows more detailed morphology analysis of an individual against a control model (built based on [10]). Figure 4 (lower right) gives a preliminary but interesting example (red represents expansion, blue indicates compression). The difference image is created by calculating the point to point displacement from an individual to the control model. It can be seen clearly that the eyes are smaller (a strong FAS indicator), while the lip regions are similar to the normal (green represent neutral deformation). This first proves the complexity of FAS discrimination as there is no golden standard that is applicable to all. Further, it calls for the need to build more bespoke control models (e.g. based on ethnic background) which is a natural extension our current work.

Table 1. Accuracy of different models. 'Param No.' is the number of parameter in millions. Euc Dic is the mean Euclidean distance between the GT and the prediction in 2D. Norm-err 3D is the percentage of normalized error distance calculated in 3D. 'PFL err' stands for the PFL measurement error in millimeters.

Model	Param No.	2D Euc Dis	Norm-err 3D	PFL err (mm)
$\mathcal{RB}$	5.9	12.7 ± 17.3	45.8 ± 51.2	22.8 ± 19.6
$\mathcal{HM_V}$	1.8	0.76 ± 0.70	5.1 ± 4.4	1.4 ± 1.1
$\mathcal{HM_S}$	3.6	0.78 ± 0.72	5.3 ± 4.6	1.6 ± 1.3
$Ours$	0.6	$\mathbf{0.67 \pm 0.63}$	$\mathbf{4.3 \pm 3.9}$	$\mathbf{1.2 \pm 0.8}$

---

[2] It is possible to calculate $|\cdot|_2$ using Geodesic distance, we choose Euclidean distance here to match the normalization factor–the inter-ocular distance, which is calculated using Euclidean distance.

To conclude, we have presented a fully automatic landmark detection method to facilitate facial analysis and FAS detection of infants. As no human intervention is required, the method reduces the time burden and human effort greatly and facilitates analysis of larger populations in the future.

References

1. British Medical Association, et al.: Alcohol and pregnancy: preventing and managing fetal alcohol spectrum disorders, February 2016
2. Douglas, T.S., Mutsvangwa, T.E.: A review of facial image analysis for delineation of the facial phenotype associated with fetal alcohol syndrome. Am. J. Med. Genet. Part A **152**(2), 528–536 (2010)
3. Wu, Y., Ji, Q.: Facial landmark detection: a literature survey. Int. J. Comput. Vis. **127**, 115–142 (2018)
4. Qi, C.R., Su, H., Mo, K., Guibas, L.J.: PointNet: deep learning on point sets for 3D classification and segmentation. In: Proceedings of the IEEE Conference on Computer Vision and Pattern Recognition, pp. 652–660 (2017)
5. Yi, L., Su, H., Guo, X., Guibas, L.J.: SyncSpecCNN: synchronized spectral CNN for 3D shape segmentation. In: Proceedings of the IEEE Conference on Computer Vision and Pattern Recognition, pp. 2282–2290 (2017)
6. Le, T., Bui, G., Duan, Y.: A multi-view recurrent neural network for 3D mesh segmentation. Comput. Graph. **66**, 103–112 (2017)
7. Buolamwini, J., Gebru, T.: Gender shades: intersectional accuracy disparities in commercial gender classification. In: Conference on Fairness, Accountability and Transparency, pp. 77–91 (2018)
8. Toshev, A., Szegedy, C.: DeepPose: human pose estimation via deep neural networks. In: Proceedings of the IEEE Conference on Computer Vision and Pattern Recognition, pp. 1653–1660 (2014)
9. Newell, A., Yang, K., Deng, J.: Stacked hourglass networks for human pose estimation. In: Leibe, B., Matas, J., Sebe, N., Welling, M. (eds.) ECCV 2016. LNCS, vol. 9912, pp. 483–499. Springer, Cham (2016). https://doi.org/10.1007/978-3-319-46484-8_29
10. Suttie, M., et al.: Facial dysmorphism across the fetal alcohol spectrum. Pediatrics **131**(3), e779–e788 (2013)
11. Nibali, A., He, Z., Morgan, S., Prendergast, L.: Numerical coordinate regression with convolutional neural networks. arXiv preprint arXiv:1801.07372 (2018)

A Device-Independent Novel Statistical Modeling for Cerebral TOF-MRA Data Segmentation

Baochang Zhang[1,2], Zonghan Wu[1,2], Shuting Liu[3],
Shoujun Zhou[1(✉)], Na Li[1,2], and Gang Zhao[4]

[1] Shenzhen Institutes of Advanced Technology, Chinese Academy of Sciences,
Shenzhen, China
sj.zhou@siat.ac.cn
[2] Shenzhen Colleges of Advanced Technology, University of Chinese Academy
of Sciences, Shenzhen, China
[3] School of Graduate School at Shenzhen, Tsinghua University,
Shenzhen, China
[4] Neurosurgery Department, General Hospital of Southern Theater Command,
PLA, Guangzhou, China

Abstract. Among the model-driven segmentation methods, the Maximum a Posterior (MAP) & Markov Random Field (MRF) is the popular statistical framework. However, there remains a dominating limitation in the existing statistical modeling, i.e., the data imaged by MR scanners with different types and parameters cannot be adaptively processed to lead accurate and robust vessel segmentation, as is well-known to the researchers in this field. Our methodology steps contribute as: (1) a region-histogram standardization strategy is explored to the time-of-flight magnetic resonance angiography data; (2) a Gaussian mixture models (GMM) is constructed with three Gaussian distributions and a knowledge-based expectation-maximization algorithm is explored to obtain the GMM parameters; (3) a probability feature map is captured according the estimated vascular distribution weight in GMM and then is embedded into the Markov high-level process to relieve the label field noise and rich the vascular structure. Our method wins out the other models with better segmentation accuracy and the sensibility to small-sized vessels or large arteriovenous malformation mass, which is validated on three different datasets and obtains satisfying results on visual and quantitative evaluation with Dice similarity coefficient and positive predictive value of 89.12% and 95.66%.

Keywords: Cerebrovascular segmentation · Statistical model · Markov Random Field · Data standardization · Probability feature map

This work was funded by the National Natural Science Foundation of China (No. 81827805), National Key R&D Program of China (No. 2018YFA0704102) and supported by the Key Laboratory of Health Informatics in Chinese Academy of Sciences, and also by Shenzhen Engineering Laboratory for Key Technology on Intervention Diagnosis and Treatment Integration.

H. Greenspan et al. (Eds.): CLIP 2019/UNSURE 2019, LNCS 11840, pp. 172–181, 2019.
https://doi.org/10.1007/978-3-030-32689-0_18

1 Introduction

Cerebrovascular segmentation is significant to present the three-dimensional (3D) structure of cerebral vessels and is beneficial to clinical diagnosis and treatment process. Traditional segmentation mainly depends on the manual operation of clinicians, which has the disadvantages of poor reproducibility and low efficiency. Recently, Deep-learning methods [1] realized the optimal segmentation on many medical image analysis tasks, while it is very hard to obtain vascular ground-truths (GT) from complex image context. High-efficient statistical modeling benefits not only clinicians but also deep-learning enthusiasts. Thus, it is our main research motivation.

For cerebrovascular segmentation from Time-of-flight Magnetic Resonance Angiography (TOF-MRA) data, Moccia et al. [2] completely reviewed the existing segmentation methodology, including active contour model, threshold-based segmentation, Hessian-matrix based model, and statistical model. The last two methods draw our recent interest in developing a more accurate and robust model.

Hessian-Matrix Based Model: It is often used to differentiate and enhance the ball-, tube-, and plane-like structures with the analysis of the second-order intensity derivatives or the Hessian-matrix eigenvalues. Hessian-based feature, i.e., eigenvalues and eigenvectors have been designed to construct a few of vessel functions by some researchers [3]. Especially, the recent vessel function proposed by Jerman et al. [4] presents satisfying contrast and the ratio of signal to noise on the resultant filtering response image. Although Hessian-matrix based model highlights the vessel-like object, it cannot directly lead an accurate segmentation.

Statistical Model: An adaptive algorithm for cerebrovascular segmentation from TOF-MRA data is proposed by Wilson and Noble [5], where the finite mixture models (FMM) is a weighted combination of two Gaussian distributions and a uniform one. Wen et al. [6] split FMM into a Rayleigh distribution and two Gaussian ones. However, they did not consider the neighborhood constraint around a voxel, which resulted in vascular fragments and pseudo-vessels. Hassouna et al. [7] employed Maximum a Posterior & Markov random field (MAP-MRF) to relieve the FMM-processing noise and keep the segmentation continuity. Zhou et al. [8] further enriched the vascular structure by using statistical modeling on MAP–MRF and multi-pattern neighborhood system.

The above statistical methods only make limited improvement on their designated experimental dataset. As far as we know, no one has proposed a self-adapting statistic model to segment cerebral vessel in the TOF-MRA data from MR equipment with different scanner-types, imaging parameters, and individual difference of patients.

Our work contributes to the challenge in four aspects. Firstly, we present an efficient data standardization strategy to make the algorithm focus on the region without a skull, which helps statistic model adapt to segment cerebral vessel in the TOF-MRA data from anywhere and any patients. Secondly, a knowledge-based expectation maximization (EM) algorithm is proposed to estimate the Gaussian mixture models (GMM) parameters, which helps to obtain better parameters of the vascular distribution. Thirdly, the vascular probability feature map is extracted and a novel neighborhood energy function for MRF is obtained to further improve the segmentation performance. Lastly, our method is validated on three different datasets (total of 139 clinical data). Due to data being influenced by different factors, such as scanners, imaging parameters, and patients, our proposed method greatly improves the Dice similarity coefficients by 7.15%–38.20% and improves the sensitivity by 9.45%–48.41% than the existing methods. In terms of vascular network coverage, and environmental complexity, the visual comparison in between our method with the above traditional methods are shown in Fig. 1.

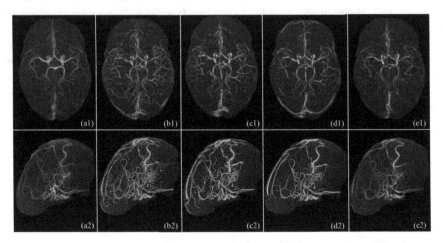

Fig. 1. The cerebrovascular segmentation results using different methods. The maximum intensity projections of the TOF-MRA without skull (a1 ∼ a2). Subfigures (b–e) are the segmentation results of the proposed method, Zhou's [8], Lu's [9], and Wilson and Nobel [5].

2   Method

The proposed method consists of four steps: (1) data standardization; (2) GMM and initialization; (3) GMM parameters estimation using knowledge-based EM algorithm; (4) a novel neighborhood constraint energy function for MAP-MRF.

2.1   Data Standardization

As a fact, most of cerebrovascular voxels distribute in the middle and high intensity, and the proportion of cerebrovascular voxels in intracranial volume is relatively small (about 1% ∼ 5%). Another fact comes from numerous experiential validations. Namely, GMM accuracy is mostly dominated by the non-vascular region, whereas little by fitting the vascular regions. The existing methods often modeled the whole data space of original TOF-MRA data, where the non-vascular region inevitably facilitates the fitting errors and computational redundancy. In this respect, skull-stripping step is necessary, for which we use the FSL-BET [10] tool to greatly reduce the non-vascular region and stabilize the histogram of intracranial volume.

To improve the robustness, the histogram specification is employed to reduce the difference of the histograms of various TOF-MRA data. We use the proposed method without histogram specification to process all the TOF-MRA data. Then we select a TOF-MRA data that has the best visual vessel segmentation result and regard its intensity distribution as the specific histogram. After that, we standardize the histogram of the other TOF-MRA data to the specific histogram. Since discrete transformation may have a one-to-many relationship, a $3 \times 3 \times 3$ Gaussian kernel (commonly used with an empirical variance of 0.4) is used to convolve with the TOF-MAR data, which increases the vascular intensity continuity as shown in Fig. 2.

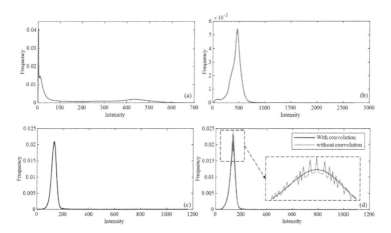

Fig. 2. The process of data standardization illustrates the resultant histograms of (a) the original TOF-MRA data; (b) skull-stripped data; (c) the specific one and (d) the transformed one.

2.2 GMM and Initialization

After data standardization, the resultant intensity distribution (shown in Fig. 2-a) facilitates to divide the voxels of skull-stripping data into one vessel class (cerebral vasculature) and two background classes (brain tissues and cerebrospinal fluid). Therefore, we use two Gaussian distributions to model the background classes, and another one for the vessel class, namely

$$\begin{cases} M(y) = \sum_{i=1}^{3} w_{Gi} f_{Gi}(y|u_i, \sigma_i) \\ \sum_{i=1}^{3} w_{Gi} = 1 \\ f_{Gi}(y|u_i, \sigma_i) = \frac{1}{\sqrt{2\pi}\sigma_i} exp\left(\frac{-(y-u_i)^2}{2\sigma_i^2}\right) & i \in [1, 2, 3] \end{cases} \quad (1)$$

where the functions $f_{Gi}(y|u_i, \sigma_i)(i = 1, 2, 3)$ are Gaussian distributions; $f_{G3}(y|u_3, \sigma_3)$ corresponds to the cerebrovascular region; $f_{G2}(y|u_2, \sigma_2)$ corresponds to the gray and white matters; $f_{G1}(y|u_1, \sigma_1)$ corresponds to cerebrospinal fluid and lateral ventricle; $w_{Gi}(i = 1, 2, 3)$ are the weights of these categories; y is the observed intensity of each voxel in TOF-MRA data. K-means algorithm is used to initialize the GMM parameters using three points (i.e., a quarter of the peak value, peak value, and twice peak value) as the start points. The curve line of the GMM initialization is shown in Fig. 3-b.

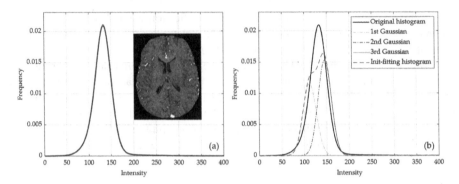

Fig. 3. After data standardization, the intensity of skull-stripped TOF-MRA data (a) and the initial curve line of GMM (b).

2.3 Knowledge-Based EM Algorithm for GMM Parameters Estimation

As we all know, the proportion of non-vascular voxels is much larger than that of cerebrovascular voxels in whole TOF-MRA volume, which will make the EM algorithm unable to estimate the parameters of vascular distribution fairly. Hence, we collect some vascular points using region growing algorithm, which would provide some knowledge for estimating vascular distribution. Then all the voxels D of skull-stripped volume are divided into un-labeled and labeled voxels (i.e., D_u and D_l). To make full use of labeled data and better fit the vascular distribution, a knowledge-based machine learning algorithm is used to estimate the GMM parameters and is iteratively updated as follows.

$$[u_i]_{k+1} = \frac{\sum_{y_j \in D_u} [p(G_i|y_j)]_k y_j + \sum_{y_j \in D_{li}} y_j}{\sum_{y_j \in D_u} [p(G_i|y_j)]_k + N(D_{li})} \tag{2}$$

$$[\sigma_i^2]_{k+1} = \frac{\sum_{y_j \in D_u} [p(G_i|y_j)]_k (y_j - [u_i]_k)^2 + \sum_{y_j \in D_{li}} (y_j - [u_i]_k)^2}{\sum_{y_j \in D_u} [p(G_i|y_j)]_k + N(D_{li})} \tag{3}$$

$$[w_i]_{k+1} = \frac{\sum_{y_j \in D_u} [p(G_i|y_j)]_k + N(D_{li})}{N(D)} \tag{4}$$

where D_{li} is the labeled dataset of the ith distribution. $N(\cdot)$ is the number of voxels in the given set. According to Bayesian criterion, the posterior probability $p(G_i|x_j)$ is calculated by:

$$p(G_i|y_j) = \frac{w_{Gi} f_{Gi}(y_j|u_i, \sigma_i)}{\sum_{i=1}^{3} w_{Gi} f_{Gi}(y_j|u_i, \sigma_i)} \tag{5}$$

According to the maximum a posteriori (MAP) classification, if a voxel y_j meets $p(G_3|y_j) - max\{p(G_i|y_j); i = 1, 2\} > 0$, we infer it to be a vascular point initially.

2.4 Neighborhood Constraint with Vessel Prior

Probability Feature Map. Hessian-based multi-scale filter [4] highlights the tubular structure and suppress background efficiently, but its filtering response cannot represent the probability of vessels. Without loss of generality, we facilitate the filtering response to be probabilistic using estimated GMM parameters. The probability feature map V_f is defined as:

$$V_f(v) = \frac{1}{1 + \left(\frac{\tau}{v}\right)^2} \tag{6}$$

where v is multi-scale filtering response, and the parameter τ is obtained by solving the following equations:

$$\aleph(\tau) = w_{G3} \int_V 1 dv; \ \aleph(\tau) = \int_\tau^1 \int_V \varepsilon(v, \tau) dv d\tau; \ \varepsilon(v, \tau) = \begin{cases} 1 & v \geq \tau \\ 0 & v < \tau \end{cases} \tag{7}$$

where w_{G3} is the estimated weight of the vascular Gaussian distribution in Eq. (1), and $\aleph(\tau)$ presents the number of voxels that meet the condition. Figure 4 shows the obvious difference between the probability feature map and the multi-scale filtering response.

Neighborhood Constraint. In this study, we organize the novel six-neighborhood energy function by GMM process result and probability feature map. The new potential energy function $U(x_r, r)$ comes from two parts, not only comes from the initial label field obtained by GMM corresponding to $\varphi_1(x_r, x_{r^*})$, but also comes from probability feature map corresponding to $\varphi_2(V_{f_r}, V_{f_{r^*}})$, which is defined as:

$$U(x_r, r) = \sum_{r^* \in \eta_r} (\alpha_1 \varphi_1(x_r, x_{r^*}) + \alpha_2 \varphi_2(V_{f_r}, V_{f_{r^*}})) \tag{8}$$

where r is the index of a point and $r^* \in \eta_r$ is the index around six-neighborhood. where x_r, x_{r^*} takes a value from the label set $L = \{L_v, L_b\}$ with L_v and L_b being the vessel class and the background class, respectively. V_{f_r} is the value of the rth position in a probability feature map. Given that scale factors meet $\alpha_1 + \alpha_2 = 1$, and α_1 and α_2 is set to be 0.5. $\varphi_1(x_r, x_{r^*})$ and $\varphi_2(V_{f_r}, V_{f_{r^*}})$ are defined as:

$$\varphi_1(x_r, x_{r^*}) = \begin{cases} 0, & if \ x_r = x_{r^*} \\ 1, & otherwise \end{cases} \tag{9}$$

$$\varphi_2(V_{f_r}, V_{f_{r^*}}) = |V_{f_r} - V_{f_{r^*}}| \tag{10}$$

Then, according to the MAP–MRF segmentation approach [8], the posterior probability of the vessel and background class is expressed as:

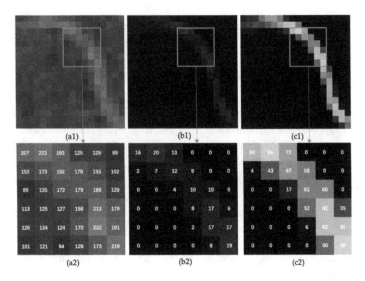

Fig. 4. Illustration of differences in between three kinds of image data with their local information on (a1) TOF-MRA data, (b1) multi-scale filtering response, and (c1) probability feature map. The subfigures in (a2 ∼ c2) show the intensity-value boards within the blue boxed region of that in (a1 ∼ c1). Note, the intensity-value in b2, c2 is multiplied by 100 for equilibrium display.

$$p(x_r = L_v|y_r) \propto f_{G3}(y_r|u_3, \sigma_3)exp(-U(x_r = L_v, r)) \tag{11}$$

And the posterior probability of the is expressed by:

$$p(x_r = L_b|y_r) \propto \frac{\sum_{i=1}^{2} w_{Gi}f_{Gi}(y_r|u_i, \sigma_i)}{\sum_{i=1}^{2} w_{Gi}} exp(-U(x_r = L_b, r)) \tag{12}$$

According to the MAP criterion, if a voxel meets $p(x_r = L_v|y_r) > p(x_r = L_b|y_r)$, we infer it to be a vascular point.

3   Experiment and Result

3.1   Materials and Implementation Environment

Our experimental materials consist of three datasets which are acquired from several MR scanners with different imaging parameters for different individuals that have healthy or diseased cerebrovascular structures. (1) MIDAS-109: 109 normal TOF-MRA datasets are collected using SIEMENS ALLEGRA 3.0T MRI scanner (TR = 35.0, TE = 3.56, flip angle = 22) from a public dataset MIDAS [11]. Each volume has the size of 448 × 448 × 128 (voxels), and the resolution is uniformly

0.51 mm × 0.51 mm × 0.80 mm. (2) AVM-20: 20 abnormal TOF-MRA datasets with arteriovenous malformation (AVM) mass, are collected using GE Signa HDx 3.0T MRI scanner (TR = 25.0, TE = 3.5, flip angle = 20) from General Hospital of Southern Theater Command of Chinese People's Liberation Army. Each volume has the size of 512 × 512 × 332 (voxels), and the resolution is uniformly 0.56 mm × 0.56 mm × 0.55 mm. (3) GZ-10: 10 normal TOF-MRA datasets are collected using GE Signa HDx 3.0T MRI scanner (TR = 30.0, TE = 3.2, flip angle = 15) from General Hospital of Southern Theater Command of PLA of China. Each volume has the size of 512 × 512 × 283 (voxels), and the resolution is uniformly 0.43 mm × 0.43 mm × 0.50 mm.

The algorithms are implemented by using MATLAB2018b, on a PC Intel® CoreTM i7-6850 k CPU @3.60 GHz*12, while the 3D visualization uses a hybrid rendering engine of VTK-8.0 with Visual Studio 2017.

3.2 Quantification Result

To make a quantitative evaluation, ten TOF-MRA data are selected from the above three datasets (Note, five from MIDAS-109, three from AVM-20, two from GZ-10). The cerebrovascular structures are manually segmented with voxel-by-voxel selections from the 10 TOF-MRA data by three neurosurgeons. The manual segmentations are treated as the ground truth to estimate the performance of models. Meanwhile, to derive a quantitative comparison of the segmentation results, three metrics are employed, *i.e.*, dice similarity coefficient $DSC = \frac{2TP}{2TP + FN + FP}$, sensitivity $Sen = \frac{TP}{TP + FN}$ and positive predictive value $PPV = \frac{TP}{TP + FP}$. where TP, FP, TN, and FN denote the voxel number of true-positive, false-positive, true-negative and false-negative results, respectively.

Our experiments consisted of four methods in three datasets, and the qualitative evaluation results are presented in Table 1. The proposed method gets an average DSC score of 89.12%, an average Sen score of 83.72%, and an average PPV score of 95.66%, which outperforms all other methods. Besides, clinical evaluation proceeded through the observations of neurosurgeons is illustrated in Table 2. Their evaluation reports were divided into three-level cases. i.e., Good, general, and poor cases according to cerebrovascular network coverage, over-segmentation, and the percentage of pseudo-vascular structures. Cerebrovascular segmentation results are shown in Fig. 1, which shows that all these methods show similar performance on the large vessel segmentation. Comparing some segmentation details, it is obvious that our segmentation result with richer vascular network coverage than all the other methods.

Table 1. The qualitative evaluation results of four different methods for three datasets

		DSC	PPV	Sen
Wilson's [5]	MIDAS-109	59.19 ± 3.2128	97.20 ± 0.7466	42.64 ± 3.3872
	AVM_20	34.12 ± 2.3709	99.28 ± 0.2875	20.62 ± 1.7375
	GZ_10	55.92 ± 5.7872	97.22 ± 0.4153	39.03 ± 5.7401
	Mean	**50.92 ± 11.6814**	**97.83 ± 1.1152**	**35.31 ± 10.3709**
Zhou's [8]	MIDAS-109	81.32 ± 3.9763	92.49 ± 2.0162	72.97 ± 7.2246
	AVM_20	81.88 ± 2.9729	93.58 ± 2.1230	72.79 ± 3.4084
	GZ_10	83.74 ± 2.0943	88.64 ± 2.5889	79.75 ± 5.8663
	Mean	**81.97 ± 3.5032**	**92.05 ± 2.8003**	**74.27 ± 6.6309**
Lu's [9]	MIDAS-109	71.09 ± 2.7068	82.30 ± 5.4044	63.31 ± 6.3041
	AVM_20	66.21 ± 1.1884	94.76 ± 1.4166	50.92 ± 1.7928
	GZ_10	61.51 ± 2.5085	90.62 ± 0.8749	46.64 ± 3.1079
	Mean	**67.71 ± 4.4080**	**87.70 ± 6.8260**	**56.26 ± 8.6423**
Our	MIDAS-109	90.93 ± 0.8302	94.80 ± 1.2320	87.39 ± 1.4320
	AVM_20	85.96 ± 4.2120	97.99 ± 1.4643	76.73 ± 6.1389
	GZ_10	89.34 ± 1.7574	94.34 ± 1.6684	85.05 ± 4.5294
	Mean	**89.12 ± 3.3068**	**95.66 ± 2.0735**	**83.72 ± 6.1810**

Table 2. Clinical evaluation of the three TOF-MRA data sets

	Avg. time	Good	General	Poor
MIDAS-109	25.71 s	97	8	4
AVM-20	73.71 s	18	1	1
GZ-10	69.67 s	8	2	0
Total		123	11	5

4 Conclusion

Our method steps contribute four parts for the MAP-MRF framework, i.e., data standardization, knowledge-based EM estimation of GMM parameters, and Markov high-level model with novel neighborhood constraint energy function, which make our proposed method more effective than the existing ones. Meanwhile, the proposed method is validated on three TOF-MRA datasets that contain 139 data totally and are acquired from different MR equipment, scanning parameters, and individuals. Extensive experimental results demonstrate that our method wins out of other ones in terms of the universality and accuracy for non-homologous TOF-MRA datasets. In addition, our method performs well on TOF-MAR data with AVM, which indicates a particular significance for computer-assisted clinical procedures. In the feature work, we will produce weak label on un-marked cerebrovascular data sets and conduct weak supervised learning, especially, we will further optimize and expand the method to automate vascular annotation and develop the deep-learning on vascular segmentation of more TOF-MRA datasets.

References

1. Zhao, F.J., et al.: Semi-supervised cerebrovascular segmentation by hierarchical convolutional neural network. IEEE Access **6**, 67841–67852 (2018)
2. Moccia, S., et al.: Blood vessel segmentation algorithms—review of methods, datasets and evaluation metrics. Comput. Methods Programs Biomed. **158**, 71–91 (2018)
3. Sato, Y., et al.: Tissue classification based on 3D local intensity structures for volume rendering. IEEE Trans. Visual Comput. Graphics **6**, 160–180 (2000)
4. Jerman, T., et al.: Enhancement of vascular structures in 3D and 2D angiographic images. IEEE Trans. Med. Imaging **35**, 2107–2118 (2016)
5. Wilson, D.L., et al.: An adaptive segmentation algorithm for time-of-flight MRA data. IEEE Trans. Med. Imaging **18**, 938–945 (1999)
6. Wen, L., et al.: A novel statistical cerebrovascular segmentation algorithm with particle swarm optimization. Neurocomputing **148**, 569–577 (2015)
7. Hassouna, M.S., et al.: Cerebrovascular segmentation from TOF using stochastic models. Med. Image Anal. **10**, 2–18 (2006)
8. Zhou, S.J., et al.: Segmentation of brain magnetic resonance angiography images based on MAP–MRF with multi-pattern neighborhood system and approximation of regularization coefficient. Med. Image Anal. **17**, 1220–1235 (2013)
9. Lu, P., et al.: A vessel segmentation method for multi-modality angiographic images based on multi-scale filtering and statistical models. Biomed. Eng. Online **15**, 120 (2016)
10. Smith, S.M.: Fast robust automated brain extraction. Hum. Brain Mapp. **17**, 143–155 (2002)
11. Bullitt, E., et al.: Vessel tortuosity and brain tumor malignancy: a blinded study1. Acad. Radiol. **12**, 1232–1240 (2005)

Three-Dimensional Face Reconstruction from Uncalibrated Photographs: Application to Early Detection of Genetic Syndromes

Liyun Tu[1](✉), Antonio R. Porras[1], Araceli Morales[2],
Daniel A. Perez[1], Gemma Piella[2], Federico Sukno[2],
and Marius George Linguraru[1,3]

[1] Children's National Health System, Sheikh Zayed Institute for Pediatric
Surgical Innovation, Washington, DC, USA
tuliyun@gmail.com
[2] Department of Information and Communication Technologies,
University Pompeu Fabra, Barcelona, Spain
[3] School of Medicine and Health Sciences, George Washington University,
Washington, DC, USA

Abstract. Facial analysis from photography supports the early identification of genetic syndromes, but clinically-acquired uncalibrated images suffer from image pose and illumination variability. Although 3D photography overcomes some of the challenges of 2D images, 3D scanners are not typically available. We present an optimization method for 3D face reconstruction from uncalibrated 2D photographs of the face using a novel statistical shape model of the infant face. First, our method creates an initial estimation of the camera pose for each 2D photograph using the average shape of the statistical model and a set of 2D facial landmarks. Second, it calculates the camera pose and the parameters of the statistical model by minimizing the distance between the projection of the estimated 3D face in the image plane of each camera and the observed 2D face geometry. Using the reconstructed 3D faces, we automatically extract a set of 3D geometric and appearance descriptors and we use them to train a classifier to identify facial dysmorphology associated with genetic syndromes. We evaluated our face reconstruction method on 3D photographs of 54 subjects (age range 0–3 years), and we obtained a point-to-surface error of $2.01 \pm 0.54\%$, which was a significant improvement over $2.98 \pm 0.64\%$ using state-of-the-art methods ($p < 0.001$). Our classifier detected genetic syndromes from the reconstructed 3D faces from the 2D photographs with 100% sensitivity and 92.11% specificity.

Keywords: Facial dysmorphology · 3D face reconstruction · 2D photography · Morphable model · Statistical shape model

1 Introduction

Over one million children are born with a genetic condition every year. Although approximately half of genetic syndromes present with facial dysmorphology, abnormal facial features are often subtle at birth and their identification by pediatricians can be

© Springer Nature Switzerland AG 2019
H. Greenspan et al. (Eds.): CLIP 2019/UNSURE 2019, LNCS 11840, pp. 182–189, 2019.
https://doi.org/10.1007/978-3-030-32689-0_19

challenging. Diagnosis delays and errors have a significant impact on the mortality and morbidity associated with genetic syndromes. As an example, the average accuracy in the detection of one of the most studied genetic syndromes, Down syndrome, by a trained pediatrician is as low as 64% in the United States [1], so methods for the early detection of genetic syndromes are critical [2].

Methods that evaluate facial dysmorphology using two-dimensional (2D) photography have shown great potential for the detection of genetic syndromes [3–5]. Due to the limitations of 2D photographs of patient faces with respect to the camera orientation and light, three-dimensional (3D) photography is preferred to quantify craniofacial dysmorphology [6–9]. However, 3D scanners are not typically available in clinics. To eliminate the dependency on expensive equipment, different works have proposed to reconstruct the 3D faces from 2D photography based on a reference template (e.g., optical-flow [10], and shape-from-shading [11]), facial landmarks fitting [12], and deep learning [13, 14]. Although these methods revolutionized 3D face reconstruction using a single image, they did not reconstruct the face boundary. A recent study [15] integrated three 2D photographs (frontal, left and right profile) of a patient for the analysis of 3D facial dysmorphology using a 3D morphable model created from 3D scans of adults. However, they did not account for 3D appearance/texture, and their reconstruction was precise only at specific sparse facial landmarks. Since the appearance is essential for accurate identification of facial dysmorphology, they used the 2D texture from one frontal 2D image at those sparse landmarks. That approach disregarded the important appearance information from the profile pictures and the role that the camera orientation plays in the texture observed in each 2D picture.

In this paper, we present a novel framework to analyze facial dysmorphology using the 3D face geometry and true appearance reconstructed from uncalibrated frontal and profile 2D photographs. First, we create a statistical shape model (SSM) of the infant face from 3D scans, which is the population that benefits most from early detection of genetic syndromes. Second, we use the geometry observed in the 2D pictures to approximate both the camera pose for each picture and the SSM parameters, which we refine using a non-linear joint optimization approach. Third, we add texture to the reconstructed 3D face by combining the observed appearance in each 2D photograph based on the camera pose with respect to the face surface. Finally, we automatically extract a set of 3D geometric and appearance descriptors, and we use them to train a classifier to identify facial dysmorphology associated with genetic syndromes.

2 Data and Methods

2.1 Data Description

We collected three independent datasets for this study. **Dataset A**: 3D photographs of 44 healthy infants for the SSM creation: 25 male and 19 female, age range 0–36 months. **Dataset B**: 3D photographs of 54 subjects including both healthy and syndromic cases for the evaluation of the face reconstruction algorithm: 34 male and 20 female, age range 3-36 months. **Dataset C**: three 2D photographs (frontal, left and right profile) of 70 subjects acquired with smartphones for evaluation of the algorithm to detect genetic syndromes: 35 male and 35 female, age range 0-36 months. Thirty-five subjects in Dataset C presented genetic syndromes (i.e. Down, Noonan, Turner, Trisomy 18, Potters, Wolf-Hirschorn syndromes, etc.), and the other 35 cases were age-, ethnicity-, and sex- matched healthy subjects. A set of facial landmarks (green dots in Fig. 1) were manually annotated for each of the 2D photographs.

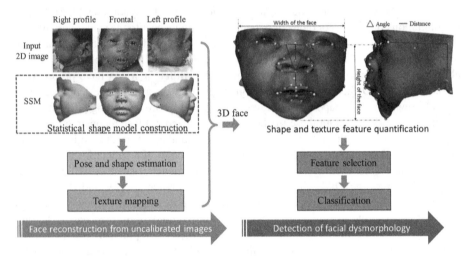

Fig. 1. Architecture of the proposed method for 3D face reconstruction and identification of facial dysmorphology associated with genetic syndromes. The green and red dots denote the anatomical landmarks correspondence between the 2D photographs and the face statistical shape model (SSM). The classification uses both shape geometry (angles and distances) and texture features (calculated around the yellow dots locations). (Color figure online)

2.2   Face Reconstruction from Uncalibrated Images

(A) Statistical Shape Model Construction. To represent a dense 3D shape of an infant's face, we created an SSM using dataset A. Each 3D scan was first mapped onto a common 2D target domain through least squares conformal mapping [16] using a subset of the sparse facial landmarks (Fig. 1) as constrains. The use of a common target domain allowed us to establish a common triangulation to re-parameterize all the 2D maps, which were then mapped back to 3D (by inverting the conformal mapping). Thus, all the original scans were re-parameterized in dense correspondence. After re-parameterization, principal component analysis was used to create the SSM of the infant face. Hence, the geometry of a face can be expressed as

$$\mathbf{V} = \mathbf{V}_0 + \sum_{i=1}^{S} b_i P_i , \tag{1}$$

where $\mathbf{V}_0 \in \mathbb{R}^{3n}$ is the mean shape of the model with n vertices, $b \in \mathbb{R}^S$ are the shape parameters, and $P \in \mathbb{R}^{3n \times S}$ are the S principal components.

Note that the goal of the above procedure is to propagate the sparse set of correspondences (at the landmark locations) to a dense set of correspondences covering the whole facial surface. Compared to other widespread approaches, such as cylindrical mapping or non-rigid iterative closest point, conformal maps have the advantage of minimizing the differential distortion between the original and re-parametrized surfaces. This is especially important when analyzing the subtle facial abnormalities of infants that are targeted in this study.

(B) Pose and Shape Estimation. We used a scaled orthographic perspective transformation to project the face SSM to the camera plane. The projected 2D position of a 3D point $v = (x, y, z)^T \in V$ from the SSM (as defined in Eq. 1) in an image plane can be written as

$$p = s\left(\begin{bmatrix} 1 & 0 & 0 \\ 0 & 1 & 0 \end{bmatrix} Rv + t\right), \tag{2}$$

where $s \in \mathbb{R}$ is the scaling, $R \in \mathbb{R}^{3 \times 3}$ is the 3D rotation matrix, and $t \in \mathbb{R}^2$ is the 2D translation in the image plane. To fit the SSM to the information observed from a 2D photograph, we minimized the projection error (E) using

$$E = \frac{1}{n} \sum_{j=1}^{n} \|q_j - p_j\|_F^2, \tag{3}$$

where q_j represents the jth 2D landmark in the image, $p_j \in p$ is the projected position of the corresponding 3D point of the SSM, and $\|.\|_F$ is the Frobenius norm. Since the optimal SSM parameters are the ones that minimize the projection error of the face geometry at each image plane, we define the following cost function

$$E = \sum_{k=1}^{3} \frac{1}{n_k} \sum_{j=1}^{n_k} \left\| q_j^k - s^k \left(IR^k v_j^k + t^k \right) \right\|_F^2, \tag{4}$$

where $v_j^k \in V_0^k + \sum_{i=1}^{S} b_i P_i^k$ represents the 3D vertices on the SSM corresponding to the jth 2D landmarks in the kth image (q_j^k), and $k \in \{1, 2, 3\}$ represents the frontal, left profile, and right profile views, respectively. I is the 2-by-3 identity matrix, and n_k is the number of landmarks used for each image. R^k, t^k and s^k represent the rotation, translation, and scaling of the kth image plane, respectively. Equation 4 was iteratively minimized using the trust-region reflective algorithm [17]. Initialized with all SSM parameters set to zero, the algorithm estimates alternately the pose (R^k, t^k and s^k) and the SSM parameters. To ensure plausibility, we constrained $b_i \in \left[-3\sqrt{\lambda_i}, 3\sqrt{\lambda_i}\right]$, where λ_i is the ith eigenvalue associated to the ith principal component in the SSM.

Since the pose and shape parameters were optimized independently, we refined our estimation by solving the following non-linear least squares problem similar to [12]:

$$\arg\min_{b_i,R^k,t^k,s^k} \left(\sum_{k=1}^{3} E^k + \delta \sum_{i=1}^{S} \left(\frac{b_i}{\sqrt{\lambda_i}} \right)^2 \right), \qquad (5)$$

where E^k is the projection error of the kth camera, $\sum_{i=1}^{S} \left(b_i/\sqrt{\lambda_i} \right)^2$ is the shape prior to ensure the plausibility of the solution, and δ is a weighting constant.

(C) Texture Mapping. To reconstruct the 3D face appearance, we computed the color L_j for each vertex v_j of the face using the following expression:

$$L_j = \sum_{k=1}^{3} w_j^k c_j^k, \qquad (6)$$

where c_j^k is the observed RGB value at the projected position of v_j in the kth image plane. The weight $w_j^k = n_j \cdot d_j^k$ is the scalar product of the normalized vector (n_j) perpendicular to the face surface at v_j and a unitary vector (d_j^k) perpendicular to the kth image plane. For each vertex, w_j^k were normalized to the sum of weights over the three images.

2.3   Detection of Dysmorphology Associated with Genetic Syndromes

(A) Feature Quantification for Shape and Texture. Both the face geometry and its appearance are relevant to detecting genetic syndromes [3, 4, 15]. To quantify geometry, we computed a set of 21 features (represented in Fig. 1), which includes distances and angles between a set of clinically meaningful facial landmarks. All horizontal and vertical distances were normalized to the width and height of the face, respectively. To quantify the facial appearance, we calculated the 3D signature of histograms of orientations (SHOT) descriptor [18] at the 14 clinically relevant landmark locations represented with yellow dots in Fig. 1. In summary, we computed a set of local histograms over eight 3D volumes defined by an isotropic spherical grid at each landmark, which was partitioned in two volumes along each of the azimuth, elevation, and radial axes. To reduce the feature dimensionality, we summarized each of the eight histograms using their average value, skewness and kurtosis [19].

(B) Classification to Detect Facial Dysmorphology. We used recursive feature elimination [20] to select the most discriminative geometric and appearance features using a linear support vector machine (SVM) classifier. Then, we evaluated the accuracy of our classifier at increasing number of features using a leave-one-out cross-validation approach. The optimal number of features was selected as the one at which the area under the receiver operator characteristic curve of the classifier converged.

3   Experimental Results

After building our SSM using dataset A, we evaluated our 3D face reconstruction algorithm using dataset B in terms of point-to-surface distances, and we compared the results with state-of-the-art methods [12–15] on the same dataset. After aligning the 3D faces of all subjects and the SSM, we projected them onto three directions to create the frontal, left and right profile images. Each projection direction was rotated with a random angle between −30 and 30° about the x, y, and z axes. Then, we reconstructed the 3D face geometry from those three views using the proposed methods. We obtained an average error of 2.01%, a significant reduction (p < 0.001 using a Wilcoxon signed-rank test) over state-of-the-art methods, as shown in Table 1. Figure 2 shows these improvements qualitatively with an example subject.

Table 1. Comparison of the average reconstruction error of the proposed method with the state-of-the-art methods. Error was normalized to the size of the face and shown in percentage.

	Bas et al. [12]	Zhu et al. [13]	Tran et al. [14]	Tu et al. [15]	Proposed
Error	3.06 ± 0.82	3.05 ± 0.96	3.73 ± 1.07	2.98 ± 0.64	**2.01 ± 0.54**

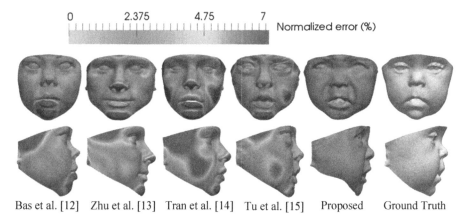

Fig. 2. Face reconstruction using different methods for an example subject. Errors are in color-code shown by comparison to the ground truth. (Color figure online)

We used our algorithm to reconstruct the 3D face geometry and appearance of the subjects from dataset C, and we evaluated our approach to detect genetic syndromes. In Fig. 3 we show two examples of the reconstructed 3D faces for one healthy subject and one infant with Down syndrome. Table 2 summarizes the classification results obtained with the proposed method using only geometry or appearance information, and the combination of these features. As we expected, the use of the reconstructed 3D appearance information that we have proposed, combined with the geometric information, obtains the best accuracy of 96.05%.

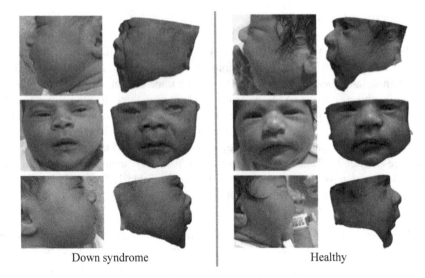

Down syndrome   Healthy

Fig. 3. Examples of the reconstructed 3D faces of a subject with Down syndrome (left) and a healthy subject (right) using the proposed method. The first column of each panel shows the uncalibrated 2D photographs, and the second column presents the 3D reconstructed faces.

Table 2. Quantitative comparative results of our approach to detect genetic syndromes.

	Accuracy (%)	Sensitivity (%)	Specificity (%)
Only geometry	81.58	84.21	78.95
Only texture	89.47	97.37	81.58
Geometry + texture	96.05	100.00	92.11

4   Conclusions

We presented a new method for accurate reconstruction of the 3D face from uncalibrated 2D photographs using a statistical shape model of the infant face. Our method achieved the lowest reconstruction error compared with state-of-the-art methods. Moreover, the proposed framework using both the 3D geometric and appearance information obtained the best accuracy to detect facial dysmorphology associated with genetic syndromes. Importantly, our framework is easily translatable to the clinics for the early detection of genetic syndromes since it only requires three uncalibrated 2D photographs of the infant's face that can be acquired using a standard mobile phone. This is important because the acquisition of calibrated photos of children is challenging, particularly for infants and children suffering from genetic disorders.

References

1. Sivakumar, S., Larkins, S.: Accuracy of clinical diagnosis in down's syndrome. Arch. Dis. Child. **89**(7), 691–693 (2004)

2. Kruszka, P., et al.: 22q11.2 deletion syndrome in diverse populations. Am. J. Med. Genet. Part A **173**(4), 879–888 (2017)
3. Zhao, Q., et al.: Digital facial dysmorphology for genetic screening: hierarchical constrained local model using ICA. Med. Image Anal. **18**(5), 699–710 (2014)
4. Cerrolaza, J.J., et al.: Identification of dysmorphic syndromes using landmark-specific local texture descriptors. In: Proceedings of IEEE International Symposium on Biomedical Imaging (ISBI), pp. 1080–1083 (2016)
5. Gurovich, Y., et al.: Identifying facial phenotypes of genetic disorders using deep learning. Nat. Med. **25**(1), 60–64 (2019)
6. Paternoster, L., et al.: Genome-wide association study of three-dimensional facial morphology identifies a variant in PAX3 associated with nasion position. Am. J. Hum. Genet. **90**(3), 478–485 (2012)
7. Weinberg, S.M., et al.: The 3D facial norms database: part 1. a web-based craniofacial anthropometric and image repository for the clinical and research community. Cleft Palate Craniofac. J. **53**(6), e185–e197 (2016)
8. Meulstee, J.W., et al.: A new method for three-dimensional evaluation of the cranial shape and the automatic identification of craniosynostosis using 3D stereophotogrammetry. Int. J. Oral Maxillofac. Surg. **46**(7), 819–826 (2017)
9. Ph, D., et al.: Cranial growth in infants—a longitudinal three-dimensional analysis of the first months of life. J. Craniomaxillofac. Surg. **46**(6), 987–993 (2018)
10. Hassner, T.: Viewing real-world faces in 3D. In: Proceedings of the 2012 IEEE Conference on Computer Vision and Pattern Recognition (CVPR), pp. 3607–3614 (2013)
11. Roth, J., et al.: Adaptive 3D face reconstruction from unconstrained photo collections. In: Proceedings of the IEEE Conference on Computer Vision and Pattern Recognition (CVPR), pp. 4197–4206 (2016)
12. Bas, A., et al.: Fitting a 3D morphable model to edges: a comparison between hard and soft correspondences. In: Asian Conference on Computer Vision (ACCV) Workshops, pp. 377–391 (2016)
13. Zhu, X., et al.: Face alignment across large poses: a 3D solution. In: Proceedings of IEEE Conference on Computer Vision and Pattern Recognition (CVPR), pp. 146–155 (2016)
14. Tuan Tran, A., et al.: Regressing robust and discriminative 3D morphable models with a very deep neural network. In Proceedings of the IEEE Conference on Computer Vision and Pattern Recognition (CVPR) (2017)
15. Tu, L., et al.: Analysis of 3D facial dysmorphology in genetic syndromes from unconstrained 2D photographs. In: Proceedings of International Conference on Medical Image Computing and Computer-Assisted Intervention. (MICCAI), 2018, pp. 347–355 (2018)
16. Lévy, B., et al.: Least squares conformal maps for automatic texture atlas generation. ACM Trans. Graph. **21**(3), 362–371 (2002)
17. Coleman, T.F., Li, Y.: An interior trust region approach for nonlinear minimization subject to bounds. SIAM J. Optim. **6**(2), 418–445 (1996)
18. Salti, S., et al.: SHOT: unique signatures of histograms for surface and texture description. Comput. Vis. Image Underst. **125**, 251–264 (2014)
19. Kim, H.-Y.: Statistical notes for clinical researchers: assessing normal distribution (2) using skewness and kurtosis. Restor. Dent. Endod. **38**(1), 52–54 (2013)
20. Guyon, I., et al.: Gene selection for cancer classification using support vector machines. Mach. Learn. **46**(1), 389–422 (2002)

Author Index

Printed in the United States
By Bookmasters